Sierra Vista Publications
P.O. Box 1899
Sierra Vista, AZ 85636

LIFESTYLE SCULPTING

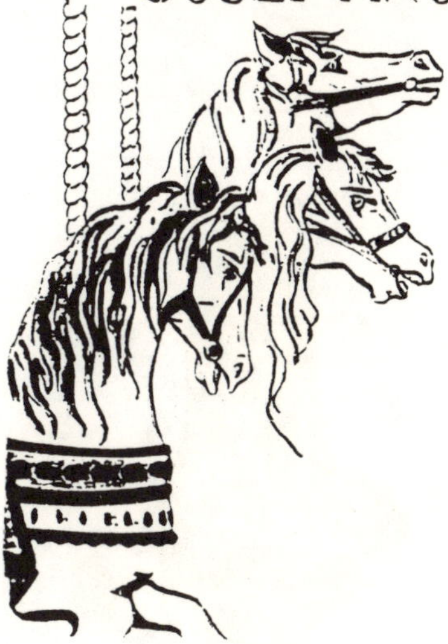

The Key to Permanent, Painless Weight Loss

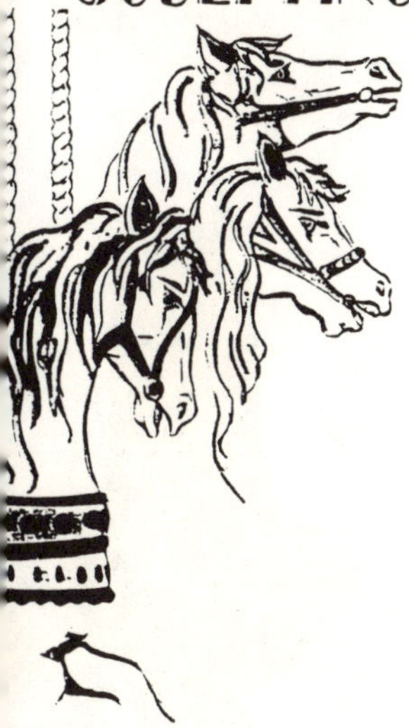

Sierra Vista Publications
P.O. Box 1899
Sierra Vista, AZ 85636

LIFESTYLE SCULPTING

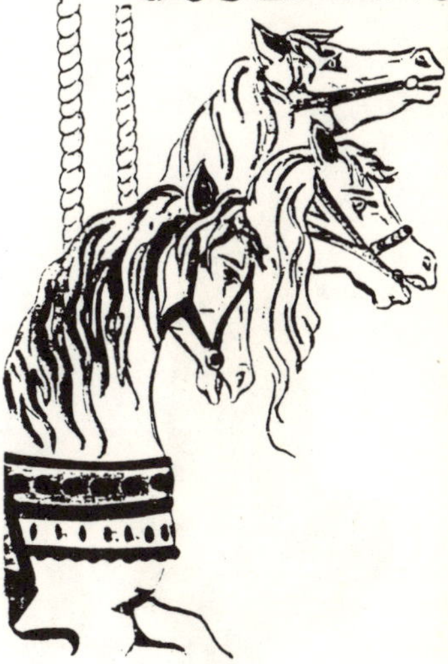

The Key to Permanent, Painless Weight Loss

Sierra Vista Publications
P.O. Box 1899
Sierra Vista, AZ 85636

LIFESTYLE SCULPTING

The Key to Permanent, Painless Weight Loss

Sierra Vista Publications
P.O. Box 1899
Sierra Vista, AZ 85636

We Want To Send You FREE Information!

Please send us your name and address so we can tell you about the books and seminars we have available.

_____ **Please place me on your mailing list.**

_____ **Please send a free sample of your newsletter, "All About Weight."**

_____ **Please send information on your Lifestyle Sculpting Seminars.**

_____ **Please send ordering information for *Lifestyle Sculpting—The Key To Permanent, Painless Weight Loss* and *Do It! Let's Get Off Our Buts.***

Name____

Address____

City ____________________________ State _________ Zip_________

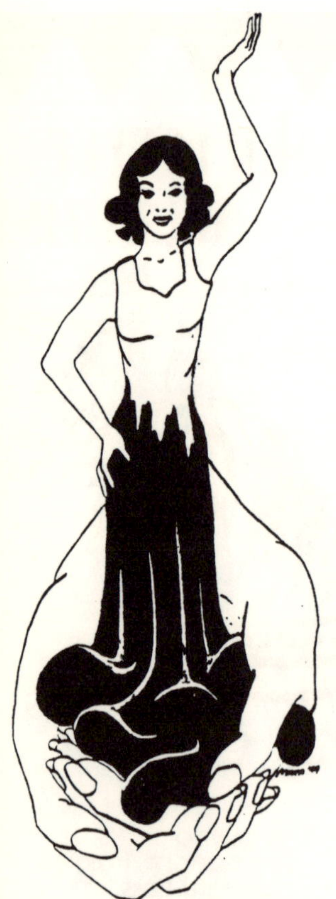

Whatever you can do or dream you can, begin it. Boldness has genius, power, and magic in it.

- W.H. Murray

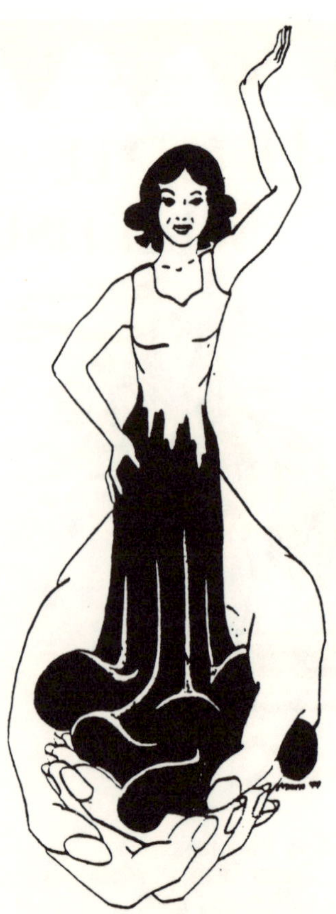

Whatever you can do or dream you can, begin it. Boldness has genius, power, and magic in it.

- W.H. Murray

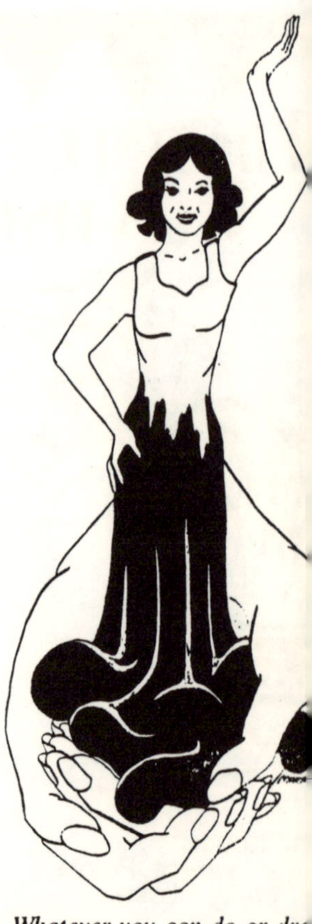

Whatever you can do or dre you can, begin it. Boldness genius, power, and magic i

- W.H. Murr

LIFESTYLE SCULPTING

The Key to Permanent, Painless Weight Loss

by

Kathleen Wells, Ph.D.

Sierra Vista Publications
Sierra Vista, Arizona

LIFESTYLE SCULPTING

The Key to Permanent, Painless Weight Loss

by

Kathleen Wells, Ph.D.

Sierra Vista Publications
Sierra Vista, Arizona

Additional copies of this book may be ordered
by sending $12.95 plus $1.00 for postage and handling
to:
Sierra Vista Publications
P.O. Box 1899
Sierra Vista, AZ 85636-1899

Library of Congress Catalog Card Number:
94-67234

ISBN 0-9642099-1-8 12.95

DEDICATION

Lifestyle Sculpting is lovingly dedicated to all those people who have known the devastation of being overweight, who have felt the pain, humiliation, and discrimination it can cause. May this program lead you to freedom and be the answer to fill your needs.

Love yourself **today**, *this instant, no matter what you weigh. Your weight has nothing whatsoever to do with who you are. You are special. You can do this. Best wishes for your liberation.*

Kathleen

Kathleen Wells

The only way to predict the future
is to have the power
to shape the future.

- Eric Hoffer

It is one of the beautiful
compensations of this life
that no one can sincerely try
to help another
without helping himself.

- Charles Dudley Warner

ACKNOWLEDGEMENTS

I would like to take this opportunity to express my sincere gratitude to those who were instrumental in helping me with this project. My appreciation goes to my longtime friend and soulmate, Mara Summers, for her wonderful illustrations and moral support through this entire process.

Additional artistic support came in the form of a lovely cover design, author's photo, and layout by Marianne Hardin, a talented artist and new friend. My thanks also go to Don Hardin for the patience and assistance he gave Marianne during the months we spent on this book.

To my husband, Robert, I extend my love and sincere thanks for patience, washed dishes, and laundry done while I sat over a keyboard, not to mention his excellent editing skills. Believe me when I say a marriage that can withstand the writing of a book is a solid one!

And to my parents and daughter, thank you for your moral support, suggestions, and encouragement.

Don't try to fly
before you have wings.

- French Proverb

AUTHOR'S NOTE

IMPORTANT INFORMATION

READ THIS BEFORE LEAPING
INTO LIFESTYLE SCULPTING!

Lifestyle Sculpting is not a diet plan nor is it an exercise plan. It does, however, encourage you to make changes in your food choices and in your activities. If you are overweight and have lead a sedentary lifestyle, *any* changes should be thought out and discussed with your physician **first**. Be sure you have no underlying medical problems of which you should be aware, before you begin making changes to a lifestyle that your body has been used to for some time. If you are under a doctor's care or on medication, this is extremely important. Do not neglect to do this.

Not everything that is faced
can be changed, but nothing
can be changed until
it is faced.

- James Baldwin

CONTENTS

All things are possible until they are proved impossible—and even the impossible may only be so, as of now.

- Pearl S. Buck

Table of Contents, *continued*

PART FOUR
SUCCESS AT LAST!

APPENDICES

LIST OF FIGURES

*Each of us really understands in
others only those feelings
he is capable of producing
himself.*

- Andre Gide

LIST OF ILLUSTRATIONS

The process of changing a
lifestyle is more important
than reaching a goal
or measuring a performance.

- Theodore Isaac Rubin

INTRODUCTION

Tell me the truth—*"**permanent** weight loss"* caught your attention, didn't it? You're probably overweight, maybe a little, maybe a lot. You're also probably a "food addict," a "compulsive eater," a "binge eater," a "yo-yoer."

You've heard all the labels. Our society loves to place labels on everyone. You've heard them and cringed—or cried. If you're all of those things, then you are just like me—or like I *was*. Oh, I'm still a compulsive eater. When the barn catches on fire, the rush of fear still sends me to the phone to call the fire department with a bag of cookies clutched to my breast. **BUT!** and this is a *huge* "but," I no longer diet, I no longer yo-yo, and I no longer weigh more than one hundred pounds above my healthy weight.

A wise man should consider
that health is the greatest
of all human blessings.

- Hippocrates

For years, I dieted, lost weight, binged, gained more weight, and dieted again. And on and on and on. You all know the cycle. Maintaining weight loss fails for many reason. I stopped the foolishness and got off the dieting carousel and so can you. I'm here to teach you how, to hold your hand, to guide you through it.

I was forty when my weight topped out at 265. I decided enough was enough. My health was failing; I couldn't walk, talk, and breathe at the same time. I sat down and thought the whole diet business over and decided there was nothing there to help me.

Thoroughly frustrated with what was available to me, I devised two plans of my own. They worked, and most of my weight has stayed off for more than three years. Hold on now. That doesn't mean I've regained part of what I lost. It means the weight I lost first has been gone for several years. The rest of the weight has come off gradually since that initial loss three years ago and none of it has come back. In these pages, I will share with you the plans that have allowed me to do this.

When the student is ready,
the teacher appears.

- Author Unknown

One of the plans is *Lifestyle Sculpting* and the other is the STOP Plan. You will enjoy using this program because you will eat what you want, when you want, and you won't feel guilty. You won't feel guilty because you will have made a *conscious choice* to eat. If you fully embrace the *Lifestyle Sculpting* and STOP Plans, they will be the last programs you will ever need to lose weight and to maintain your weight loss. This program offers real choices for real people. Male or female, young or old, Life*style Sculpting* **will** work for you. This program will last you a lifetime.

You may have jumped to some conclusions about what this book is all about when you saw the reference to weight loss in the title. Let me tell you what this book *isn't*. It isn't another useless diet book. You won't find charts to keep track of your weight loss or exercise days. You won't find a list of food choices and forbidden foods. None of these things offer *permanent* weight loss *unless* you do them ***forever.***

Do you want to pay attention to exactly what you eat every minute of every day, ***foreve*r**? **I** don't. I have more important things to think about, and

As a man thinketh so is he, and as a man
chooseth so is he.

- Ralph Waldo Emerson

I'll bet you do too. Do you want to jog three miles a day, every day, ***forever?*** I don't—and I didn't.

Permanent weight loss comes from one thing—a change in your lifestyle. If yours is like mine was, you are acquainted with the lifestyle and eating habits from hell. These have to be exorcised from your day-to-day existence if you ever hope to achieve permanent weight loss. Oh, they'll slip back into your life once in a while. You will even *let* them in on purpose for special occasions or when the comfort food is more important to you than the weight loss, but you will only do this when you *choose* to do so. We all make choices.

Now, wait a minute. I saw your hackles rise from here. No, for the compulsive eater, weight loss is not a matter of having will power, no matter what thin friends, family, or physicians tell you. It isn't a matter of deciding to drop twenty pounds and going from real soda to diet soda. It is a *real* problem, a very serious problem.

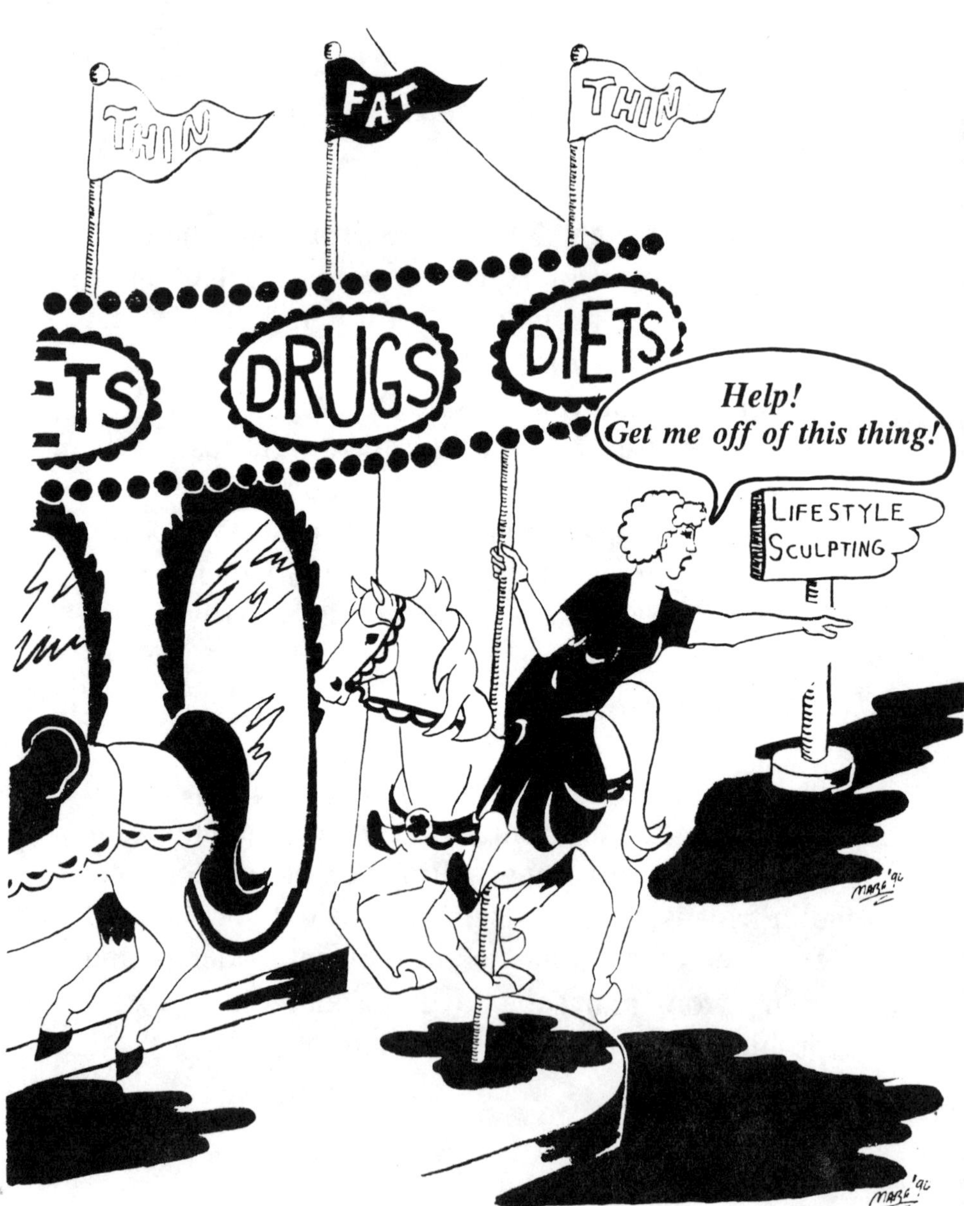

DIETING CAROUSEL

Obesity is an eating disorder of the most insidious kind. Insidious because it becomes a vicious cycle. You eat for whatever your personal reasons (we'll look closely at those), then your self-esteem drops. That makes you unhappy and insecure and you eat more, making you more unhappy and so on. Then the second vicious cycle begins, with you dieting, losing, gaining more, dieting, losing, and gaining yet again. Insidious or not—you **can** beat it. You can get off that dieting carousel forever. I did. It is up to you. I will teach you what you need to know to make your choice.

Lifestyle Sculpting is all about choices and options. We all have them; we all exercise them. *Lifestyle Sculpting* gives you credit for having common sense and the ability to use moderation.

The STOP Plan in this book will teach you how to educate yourself to your own personal demons. You will learn to guard against them, to control them, to choose when to let them in, and when you do, you will do so without guilt or remorse. The next time you eat a carton of Mocha Almond Delight ice cream, you will have *chosen* to do so

Although the world is full
of suffering,
it is also full of the
overcoming of it.

- Helen Keller

after thinking it through, considering your options and consequences, and making a deliberate choice. By using *Lifestyle Sculpting* and the STOP Plan, most of the time you won't eat the food you just picked up. You might get it out, might taste it, or even have a small serving, but most of the time you'll choose to put it back in the depths of your freezer for the enjoyment of those wicked, slender traitors in your family—and you will feel *wonderful* about it!

Let *Lifestyle Sculpting* teach you how to educate yourself about the things you need to know to win the weight loss battle once and for all. Then practice the STOP Plan as it is taught here, for a lifetime of making healthy choices and being happy **today**, no matter *what* you weigh.

The result will be a healthy, happy you who will gradually lose weight and become a free person without diets, drugs, gimmicks, or regulated exercise. Let *Lifestyle Sculpting* be the last book about weight loss you ever buy. Join me now to begin a lifetime of freedom from obesity and compulsive eating. Join me ***today***, won't you?

Resolve to find thyself; and to know that he who finds himself, loses his misery.

- Matthew Arnold

PART ONE

Recognition And Acceptance

Defining Your Personal Overweight Problem

A man cannot be comfortable without his own approval.

- Mark Twain

CHAPTER ONE

Are You Really Overweight?

Self-reverence, self-knowledge, self-control, these three alone lead life to sovereign power.
- Lord Alfred Tennyson

The title of this chapter may seem like a silly question from a book about weight. After all, you wouldn't be contemplating spending money on a book about weight loss if you didn't have a weight problem, right? ***Wrong***. How many of you have known someone in perfect condition who considered herself or himself a blimp? If you haven't known someone like this personally, you are at least aware of the problem. I am sure you have all seen the stories about bulimic and anorexic women. People occasionally have trouble differentiating between being slightly overweight, overfat, truly obese, or just unhappy with their appearance.

Mockery is often the result of a poverty of wit.

- Jean de La Bruyere

I have known the true meaning of being morbidly obese. I suspect many of you have as well. Surprisingly, many do not understand what it really means to be obese. This is especially true of those lucky family members, neighbors, associates, and physicians who are thin. Of course, you and I are talking about being too heavy or too fat as seen on a bathroom scale or in the too-tight fit of our clothing. But it is necessary to separate those who truly have a problem from those who suffer from body hate syndrome.

What are the elements of being overweight? Does overweight only show on the scale or in tight clothing? Of course not. It includes emotions, feelings. Feelings of humiliation, discrimination, and personal frustration. It includes tasks that, to a slim person, are second nature. Difficult situations like finding clothes that fit comfortably, being unhealthy, and being given impossible tasks by those we respect or love.

The most important aspect of being overweight is, of course, being unhealthy. How many of you can walk several blocks to work or at the mall without getting winded? Without your feet, knees, or back

Our entire life, with our fine moral code and our precious freedom, consists ultimately in accepting ourselves as we are.

- Jean Anouilh

hurting? A flight of stairs? You have to be kidding! Do you gasp like a fish out of water, your heart pounding like a jackhammer, after hurrying to catch a bus? Maybe your health issues are not so blatant. Tired all the time? Catch every cold and flu bug that flies by? Sounds like you have a problem—a fat problem—a *lifestyle* problem.

Humiliation. Ah, this is a *big* one. Those of us who have known morbid obesity or even moderate overweight have felt this from time to time. You know the feeling. One airline seat is barely enough for just you. Fellow passengers watch in disgust as you try to maneuver down a narrow aisle and into a seat suitable for a pygmy. Lawn chairs or toilet seats snap under your weight. You blame faulty construction and not your weight.

Ladies, you see your doctor because you're allergic to nylon—you ***must*** be. You keep getting sores on the inside of your thighs where they rub together when you wear pantyhose!

Discrimination doesn't exist in this country, right? We've come a long way, baby? **Wrong!** A big

Here's A Hint

We all need an imaginary garbage can into which we can toss useless things. Later in the book we'll talk about some of the wasteful things that will go into the can. Here's the first thing you can toss into it before slamming the lid! Get it into your head, if it isn't already, that thin people will never completely understand what you are going through. They may sincerely try, they may come close, but they will never be able to completely grasp what we have felt because they haven't experienced it firsthand. So when they give you these impossible things to do, when they say things that are hurtful, toss the pain in the can and *slam the lid on it*. As you get better, you can educate the important thin people in your life to offer you support and understanding. The ones who won't try or just can't get it, who can't develop some understanding—forget them, they aren't worth your efforts. Focus your energy on you and get going. You can do this and end those frustrating experiences! ***Do it today!***

wrong, bull pucky, no way, not true! Ever been turned down for a job for which you are highly qualified because you were "portly"? Oh, they won't admit it, they'd get sued from here to hell and back, but you know it—you *feel* it.

How about eating in restaurants where the maitre d' puts you at a table by the kitchen and behind a potted rubber plant? And then, when you eat, you feel the stares of other patrons as they judge you and what's on your plate.

Then there are the trips to the grocery store. Do people take surreptitious looks into your cart to see what you're buying? You can feel their disapproval over that ice cream you purchased for your skinny husband and your kids, while they envision *you* stuffing it in your face.

Clothes and services? Few companies consider overweight people. Only recently have a plethora of catalogs, carrying attractive clothing for large individuals come about. Before that, the women wore tents—you remember—those drapes euphemistically called muu-muus.

Don't let life discourage you.
Everyone who got where he is
had to begin where he was.

- Richard L. Evans

They had huge, brightly colored flowers all over them as if that would make us more inconspicuous! And you men bought your clothes at the Big and Tall stores. A "real" department store didn't carry anything to fit you. Chairs in doctor's offices or shops are never far enough apart to handle our derrieres, so we lap over onto the seat next to us and set our coats across our hips to hide the fact that we take up one and a half chairs.

And impossible tasks? We all know those. The doctor looks at your weight, gasps, and gives you orders. That's right, orders. "Eat 1,000 calories a day (never mind that you've been eating 4,000) and exercise for forty minutes a day, every day."

It also escapes his notice that you are a working mother, taking care of career and home because you *"should,"* and barely having any time to try to eat right, let alone exercise. And what about the one from your parents or spouse, "If you'd lose fifty pounds, you'd be so beautiful/handsome. You have such a pretty/attractive face." I ***hate*** that one. Thanks for *nothing*, huh?

Here's A Hint

As you assess your own overweight problem, take a good look around you. We assume, as we've been taught by society, that thin equals beautiful. But look at people you see coming and going in a busy place like a bank or an airport. What is it about the people you see who you feel are attractive that draws you to them? Is it really their weight or is it something more subtle like the tasteful clothing they have on? Or beautiful eyes? Or a genuine smile? How many of those people who attract your attention because of a nice overall appearance are thin? Not many, huh? Society may tell you that you are attracted to thin but are you really? I doubt it. I don't believe we as a culture are quite that shallow. On a recent business trip as I waited for a delayed flight, I watched the people milling about in the terminal. The attractive ones had on nice clothes, conservative make-up, and pleasant attitudes. Many were well over what would be considered a healthy weight, but they were still beautiful. Consider Elizabeth Taylor, Oprah Winfrey, and Delta Burke at their top weights. Have you ever seen anyone more drop-dead gorgeous than these women? I haven't. So think about yourself. Are you dressing as well as you can? Doing your hair or keeping it neatly trimmed? Take care of yourself and look your best no matter what you weigh. You will feel 100% better before you even begin to lose weight. Be the best you can be today and you will have the motivation you need to be better tomorrow!

Then there are those personal frustrations. Have trouble fitting into a bathtub and, even more, heaving yourself up and out of it? Do you know the feeling of not being able to cross your legs and make them stay that way? Those of us who are over forty remember Totie Fields, the overweight comedienne, who died far too young. Most of us found her hysterically funny. Most of us who have known morbid obesity personally, knew the pain she had experienced and joked about. Even as we laughed along, we cried and relived our own pain.

I hope some of you are chuckling along with me now, remembering your own "fat" experiences. I know all of these feelings, up-close and personal, as you do. Without a doubt, some of you are not laughing. The pain is too fresh, too strong. You have tears in your eyes and a fist has hold of your heart. We all know the pain of being overweight.

Now, I'm not saying that if you haven't experienced these things, you're not overweight, *but* this **is** a good place to start—a reality check, as it were.

Body Hate Syndrome

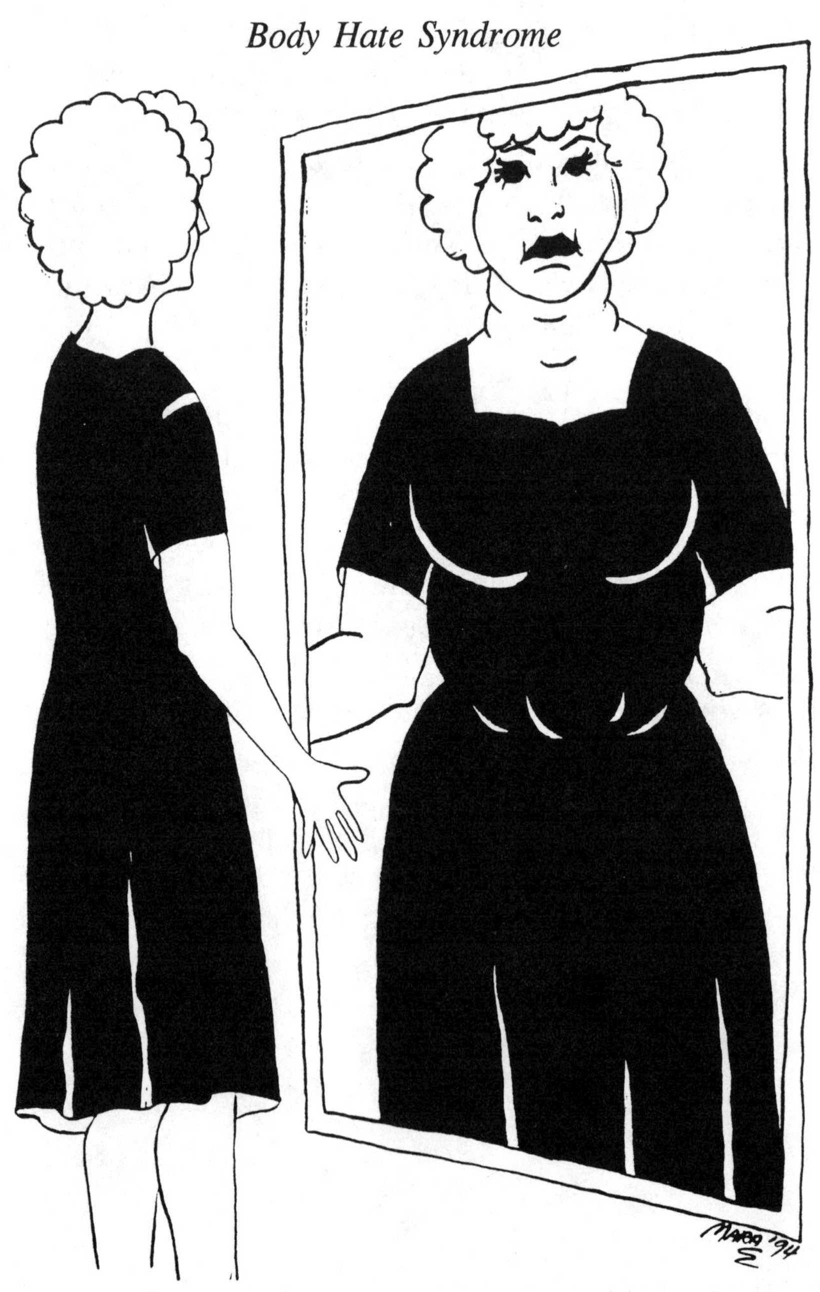

Those of you out there who believe you're too fat, take a good look at these first paragraphs. Have you ever experienced any of these things? If not, then you need to look further into your problem. For example, do your clothes really look too tight, revealing heavy thighs or rolls of fat around your middle, or do you just "feel" fat? Are you within or below the normal weight range for a person of your sex, age, and height?

Are you obsessed with how you look and terrified of gaining weight? If you answer "yes" to any of these questions, you may have a problem called Body Hate Syndrome and not have an overweight problem at all.

Body Hate Syndrome is a problem which is growing to paramount proportions in this country.

Since the issue of *Lifestyle Sculpting* is focused on those who truly need to lose weight and regain control of their lives, I will address this problem only briefly here to separate you folks from those who can benefit from *Lifestyle Sculpting*.

Our desires, once realized, haunt us again less readily.

- Margaret Fuller

Body Hate Syndrome is a psychological misconception which grows from low self-esteem and feelings of insecurity. It is an *invalid* assessment and perception of your true weight and physical condition. This often leads to serious eating disorders such as bulimia or anorexia nervosa. Sometimes these disorders are triggered by painful memories of being too heavy at one time in life, usually in early adolescence. A person with an eating disorder looks in the mirror and sees a fat person even if she or he is emaciated. For that reason, it is a good idea for everyone interested in this program to first see their doctor to get either a recommendation to proceed or an objective referral to a program specifically geared to help those with eating disorders overcome this false body image problem and become healthy again.

Now that you have seen the differences between honest overweight and a misconception of your own beauty and weight, take a long, hard look at yourself. Both problems are fixable but they do require varied strategies. If you are truly overweight—*for convenience, I will be using the term "obese" whether you are slightly overweight*

Nature never deceives us,
it is we who deceive ourselves.

- Jean Jacques Rousseau

or morbidly obese—be it by five pounds or five hundred, now is the time to leap into *Lifestyle Sculpting* and start your journey to good health. If you are not sure about the extent of your weight problem, see a physician or psychological counsellor. Physicians are always happy to tell you if they think you're too fat! Get a professional opinion of your body and *listen* to it. If you have a perception problem, seek some support and counseling to understand the problem. Life is too short to worry about being fat if you're not! Take it from those of us who really are heavy.

Those of you who are actually overweight and who can truly benefit from *Lifestyle Sculpting*, turn the page and get busy. I'm ready and waiting to show you the easy steps to successful weight loss—***permanently***.

It is better to light a candle
than curse the darkness.

- Chinese Proverb

CHAPTER TWO

What Kind Of Overweight Are You?

Theory without practice is empty; practice without theory is blind.
- Immanuel Kant

You are probably all wondering what on earth this quote has to do with weight loss, but it has been included for a very special reason. The major flaw in diets and weight loss programs is the fact that all overweight people are lumped together and treated as though obesity is caused by only one problem. This is no more effective than if an ill person went to a doctor for a cure and was given the same treatment that the doctor uses for all his patients, regardless of their individual diagnoses. It's impossible! Not all overweight people have the same problems, the same causes for their obesity. Obesity is not the disease. It is a symptom or manifestation of your own particular situation or

A theorist without practice is a tree without fruit; and a devotee without learning is a house without an entrance.

- Sa'di

condition which can range from compulsive eating to getting older to a malfunction in your physiological system. You must have a diagnosis or hypothesis on which to base your program of treatment or research. Jumping into an attempt to fix this problem, or any other, without a diagnosis is like doing research without a theory. It is unprofessional, misguided, frustrating—and worthless.

So, for *Lifestyle Sculpting* to be effective, you have to first find out what kind of overweight you are. For many of you, you already have a good idea and this will only confirm your suspicions. It may, however, point out a few other possibilities. This may be very simple, or you may be, like me, a combination of categories of overweight types. In the research I did on overweight, I defined five categories of overweight types. These are: Normal Overweights, Food-triggered Compulsives, Emotion-triggered Compulsives, Combination Compulsives, and Physiological Binge Eaters.

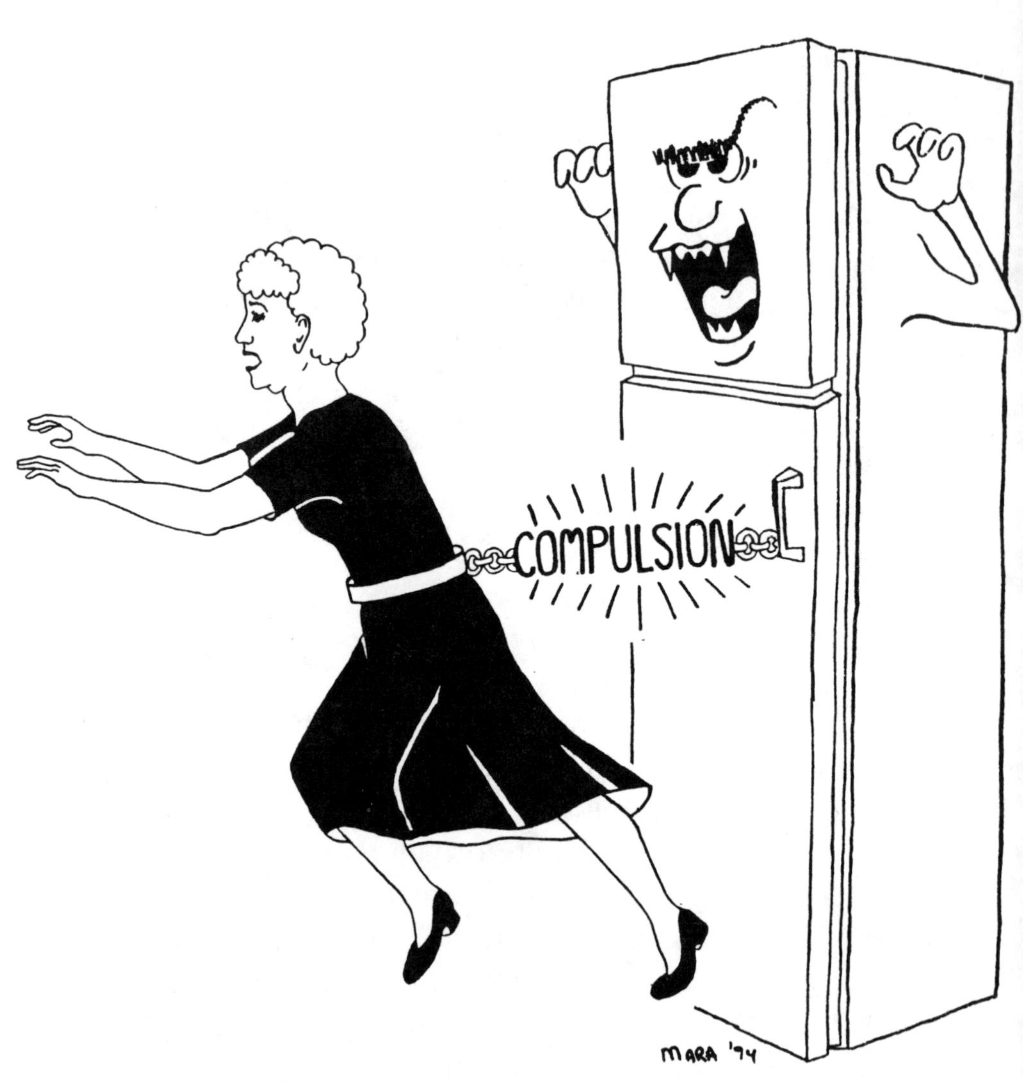
COMPULSION
MARA '94

Normal Overweights are those fortunate few—if you want to look at *any* overweight condition in those terms!—who have been thin all their lives and gained weight in response to a physiological or activity change. They may gain ten pounds after each baby or when they hit thirty and then again at forty as the metabolism slows. People with the *rare* thyroid problem would fit in this Normal Overweight category. A change from activity in high school to sitting behind a college desk or from an active job to a sedentary one will bring on a few unwanted pounds. Now as tempting as it is to want to hate these people, remember, their few pounds can be as difficult for them as a lot of weight is for you. At least we've had to deal with weight all our lives. This is a new experience for them.

Food Triggered Compulsives are people who respond to certain foods by needing to eat more. Notice I said "needing" not "wanting." This response is commonly caused by hyperinsulinemia. It is a variation in the blood sugar that sends signals to the body to increase food intake. This is often a response to high carbohydrate foods.

You May Be A Compulsive Eater if:

1. You hide Snickers Bars in your underwear drawer.

2. You eat double fudge, chocolate cupcakes straight from the freezer—while they are frozen solid.

3. You eat half-pound bacon cheeseburgers, fries, and shakes while ducked down in your car.

4. You cram your ice cream cone into your child's hand when you run into an old friend at the Dairy Queen.

The book by Drs. Heller and Heller gives excellent information on this response and a review of their book appears in the *Recommended Reading Appendix.* Not everyone responds to foods in this way, of course, but some do have a driving urge to feed their bodies shortly after eating certain foods.

For me, food triggers included refined sugars, pasta, bread, and fresh fruits. That changed somewhat when I went through the *Lifestyle Sculpting* program. I still occasionally respond to foods in this way, but it doesn't bother me as it once did. Generally, I simply avoid foods that I know will cause this kind of reaction.

Emotion Triggered Compulsives have saboteurs hiding everywhere. Being happy, sad, nervous, bored—all these and more can lead to food binges. The reasons are simple. Many of us were trained by well-meaning parents, friends, and teachers that a cookie brought relief from a skinned knee or any other pain, physical or psychological. Also, food has a certain tranquilizing effect. How many of you can stay awake after a huge Thanksgiving

If you are reluctant to ask the way,
you will be lost.

- Malay Proverb

dinner? Now, don't get all excited about dumping the blame for what you eat today on Mom. We'll discuss causation in more detail later and you'll learn that in spite of what Mom taught you twenty years ago, *you* are the one doing the food stuffing today!

Of course, many compulsive eaters are **Combination Compulsives**, triggered by both food *and* emotional factors. I certainly was. For you, the STOP Plan, coupled with the *Lifestyle Sculpting* program, is essential for weight loss. It is the only way to achieve lasting success. Now, I know it is never wise to generalize to that degree, but if weight loss and maintenance were easy and there were better solutions, would diets have a 97% failure rate? I don't think so. I believe we have been going about weight loss backwards—but I am getting ahead of myself. Let me discuss the one other type of overweight person in my research.

Physiological Binge Eaters. These folks have a difficult time ahead. They are in a good news/bad news situation. The bad news is, it is extremely

Here's A Hint

This hint is for those of you who think you might have a physiological eating problem, especially those who just cannot stop eating, ***ever.*** Contact a university in the city closest to you and get a number for their medical school and/or hospital. Call that number and ask if they have any physicians on staff who are doing research on ***Physiological Binge Eating Disorders***. If they do, make an appointment. If they don't, ask for their help in finding a university where this type of research is being undertaken. Even if you have to travel to a hospital some distance away, it is worth it. They are doing good work on this issue. You deserve help **today**.

difficult for people with a true physiological disorder to get it in hand. But the good news is, answers are being sought on this issue as we speak. This is becoming recognized by physicians as a serious, legitimate problem. Remember, this is very rare. In my research, only 1% of the overweight population even came close to being true physiological binge eaters. Do not attempt to use this disorder as an easy answer to a tough problem. It just doesn't happen that often. Binge eating disorder people have absolutely no control, ever. They can eat nonstop for several hours, spend their lives in the market or kitchen, and most probably, feel lost and hopeless. If you believe your eating goes beyond compulsive behavior, see a physician, preferably one who specializes in binge eating disorders.

Chances are you will need some medical help with your problem. Notice I said a physician who specializes in binge eating disorders. **Do not** look for a physician with a quick weight loss scheme, liquid diets, fasts, etc. Find a physician who recognizes physiological eating disorders and who does research on these problems. There are *no*

Figure One

1. Have you gained weight following the birth of a child? Y N

2. Have you ever gained weight following changes in your lifestyle, such as decreased activity due to a sedentary job, returning to school, an illness? Y N

3. If you are over thirty, do you find it easier to gain weight and more difficult to lose unwanted pounds? Y N

4. When you eat foods with refined sugars or starches, such as pasta and bread, do you crave more food a short time later? Y N

5. Do you prefer foods like bread, potatoes, and desserts over vegetables and meats? Y N

6. Have you ever sneaked food, particularly sweets, so your family/friends wouldn't know you had eaten them? Y N

7. Do you eat when you are bored, angry, upset or excited? Y N

- Continued on page 46

quick fixes—none, zero, zip, nada! So forget quick weight loss schemes.

Lifestyle Sculpting can offer even physiological binge eaters some help, of course, *but* if you truly work the program from start to finish and absolutely **cannot** make some simple changes, get help. Don't wait. Much progress is being made on these problems. You *deserve* help today.

Many of you may know just from reading these descriptions into which category you fall. If you aren't sure, or are simply curious, figure out the percentage of your lifetime you have been overweight and answer the questions in *Figure One*. Look at the answers in *Figure Two* and see how many of your answers match. Now, go to the *Obesity Diagnosis Triangle* and find your place in the scheme of things by following the example in *Figure Three*. Does the block of the triangle in which the lines intersect seem to fit your personal overweight problem? There may be some overlapping, but this should give you a basic idea of what is causing your particular problem. You

Figure One, *continued*

8. Do you "graze" or nibble constantly when you are worried? Y N

9. Do you feel guilty eating a large meal or a snack food in front of your family or out in public?
   Y N

10. Have you ever been successful at maintaining weight loss for more than a few days or weeks?
    Y N

11. At times while eating, do you feel completely out of control and unable to stop? Y N

12. Does your weight problem cause you to feel hopeless and/or depressed? Y N

13. Do you answer questions by telling people what you think they want to hear rather than what you really think? Y N

14. Do you have confidence in yourself whether you appear to be failing or succeeding? Y N

15. Do you feel equal, neither inferior nor superior, to others? Y N

Figure Two

Expected Responses to Figure One

1. Yes 2. Yes 3. Yes 4. Yes 5. Yes 6. Yes
7. Yes 8. Yes 9. Yes 10. No 11. Yes 12. Yes
13. Yes 14. No 15. No

can then focus your *Lifestyle Sculpting* on those areas of most importance to you.

In spite of the fact that we all lose weight the same way physiologically—decreased calorie or fat intake and increased activities—the importance of diagnosing your level of compulsivity is simple. By understanding the reasons for your overweight problem, you can best address what changes need to be made and how to accomplish that. Everyone can benefit from *Lifestyle Sculpting*, but you may need minor sculpting rather than a major overhaul.

If you have packed on ten pounds following the birth of a child, taking that baby on a daily walk for thirty minutes will probably do it for you. The weight will come off, and you'll get healthy while your child learns good, healthy habits from your example. For those few who have a true physiological malfunction (remember, this is *very* rare), *Lifestyle Sculpting* will help you define the level of your problem. By defining this disorder, *Lifestyle Sculpting* will encourage you to seek the help of a medical professional.

Figure Three
Obesity Diagnosis Triangle

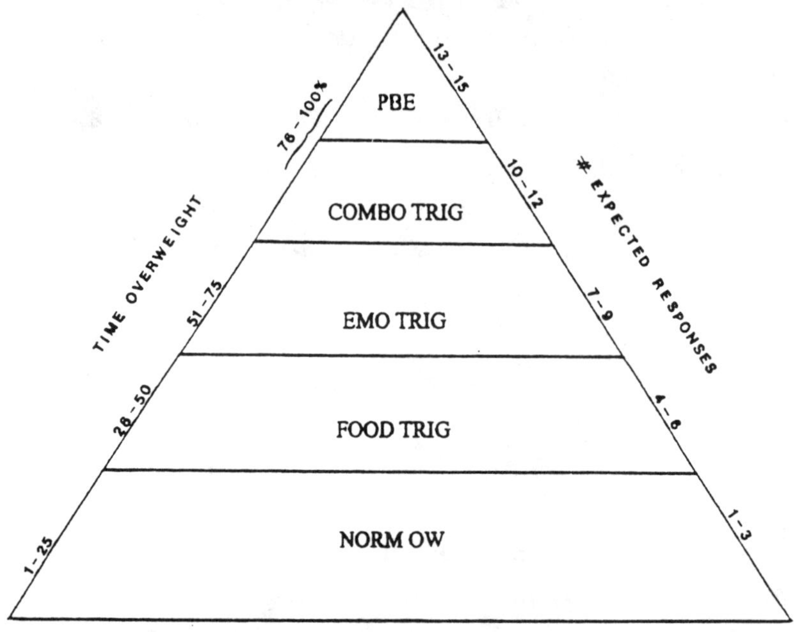

To Use:
1. Draw a line parallel to the left side of the triangle from the appropriate number of expected responses block to the bottom of the triangle.
2. Draw a line parallel to the bottom of the triangle from the appropriate time overweight block.
3. Use the obesity type (level of compulsivity) given in the block where the two lines intersect to design an appropriate intervention for weight loss.

SAMPLE:

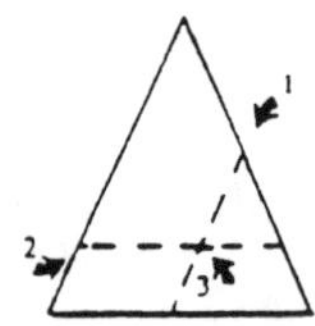

LEGEND:

PBE = Physiological binge eaters
COMBO TRIG = Combination triggers (food & emotions)
EMO TRIG = Emotional triggers
FOOD TRIG = Food triggers
NORM OW = Normal overweight

NOTE - To figure length of time overweight, divide the number of years you have been heavy by your age. Example: Age: 45. Overweight: 15 years. 15/45 = 33% of lifetime overweight.

So, go think all this through or go to the questions in *Figure One* and look at those. When you decide what your level of compulsivity is, you're ready to move on. Focus your *Lifestyle Sculpting* efforts most heavily in the areas of your own personal concern. We're all different. All overweight people are not created equal. So, let's get to it, shall we?

No one can make you feel
inferior without
your consent.

- Eleanor Roosevelt

Chapter Three

Acceptance

The future belongs to those who believe in the beauty of their dreams.

- Eleanor Roosevelt

Acceptance. A simple word, but so difficult to achieve. There are many things an overweight person must accept before she or he can move on to good health. Acceptance of self and of the situation is essential to moving forward. You must accept and then believe. Believe that you too can be healthy and happy. *Believe in your dreams.* You are worthy and your dreams are achievable.

First, it has long been accepted in substance abuse cases that the first step in healing is accepting that you have a problem. You can't fix a problem you don't think you have. So first, you have to take that hard look at yourself and say, "Yes, I am overweight. Yes, I need help." Hold on now. I know you wouldn't have picked up this book if

Don't fight your problem.
Know that there is a solution.

- Joseph Murphy

you didn't think you were overweight. But, have you accepted that you may be dependent on food physiologically and/or psychologically? If you are triggered by foods or emotions, accept that. If you look at that as a food addiction, that's okay. Most overweight people are addicted to food in one way or another. *You are not alone.*

Second, and this is an important one for permanent weight loss, you **must** accept that diets **do** work—*over and over and over.* They do what they were meant to do. They make you lose weight, quickly and *temporarily*. But, in most cases, they are not designed for long-term use and even if they were, most do not take into account the other factors needed for a lifetime of success. So accept the fact that you must **never** diet again—not for one day, one week, or one month. Not even for a special occasion to get in that exotic dress. ***NEVER!*** Diets are out, useless, passe'.

To know and yet think we do not know
is the highest attainment. Not to
know and yet think we do
is a disease.

- Lao-tzu

Now, another huge step in acceptance—*YOU ARE NOT A FAILURE.* Yes, you have undoubtedly dieted and yo-yoed for years. Yes, you're still apparently heavier than you want to be or you wouldn't be reading this. It isn't because of you; it isn't a character flaw, a lack of will power, or anything else. Every time you tried, you learned something, didn't you? Even if what you learned was that weight loss from a calorie reduction diet doesn't last. You learned the hard way about one more thing that won't work. Education of any kind is never wasted nor a failure. *Never, never, never, never!* The diets failed you; you did not fail them. You are not a bad person because the help you sought was not appropriate for you. You did the right thing by trying to lose weight to get healthy. Take what you have learned from years of losing and gaining and losing and gaining and use it to your advantage. Say enough is enough! No more diets—***ever***.

You have got to accept two more things about weight loss before it will work for you on a permanent basis. First, it took most of us a relatively long time to gain this weight and chances

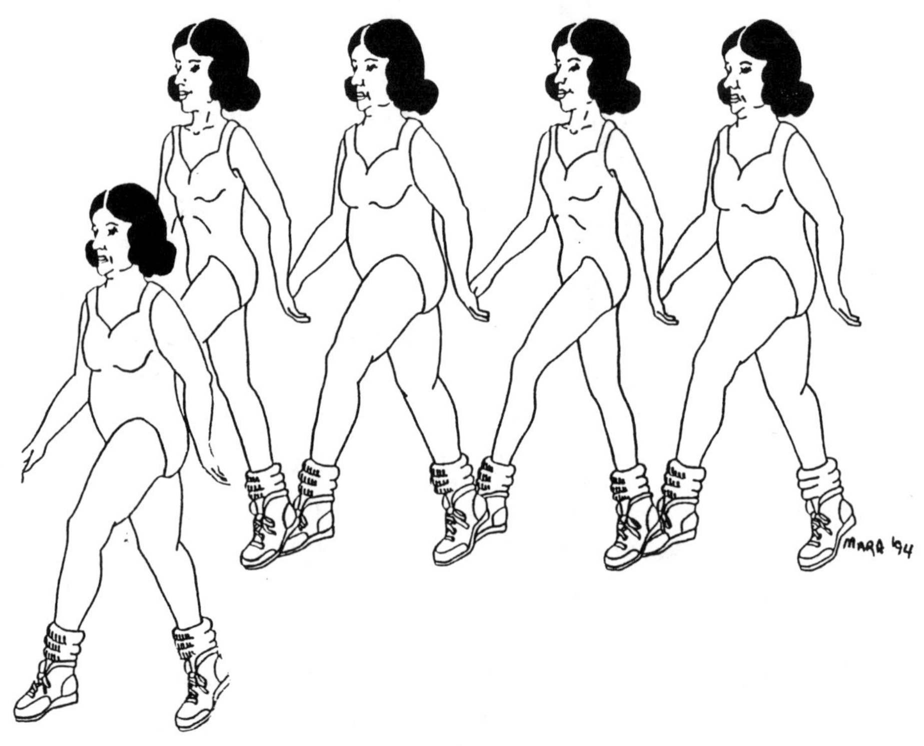

Diets DO Work—over and over and over...

are you have been heavy most, if not all, of your life. You are not going to lose this weight overnight. This may well be the most important point to accept for successful weight loss. **YOU ARE NOT GOING TO LOSE WEIGHT OVERNIGHT!** If you find some gimmick or drug that will do that for you, look out! The weight will be back quicker than ever and more of it. You sabotage your own efforts by doing this because each time you do, your body gets better and better at saving fat for starvation prevention.

That's part of the survival of the fittest that created what we, as human beings, are today. So stop looking for a quick fix. There is no such thing—none. It simply will not work and will cause more trouble later. To lose weight permanently, you must do only what you can do for the rest of your life (at least more often than not). More good days than bad, more active days than couch days. There are no two ways about it. You *will* lose weight.

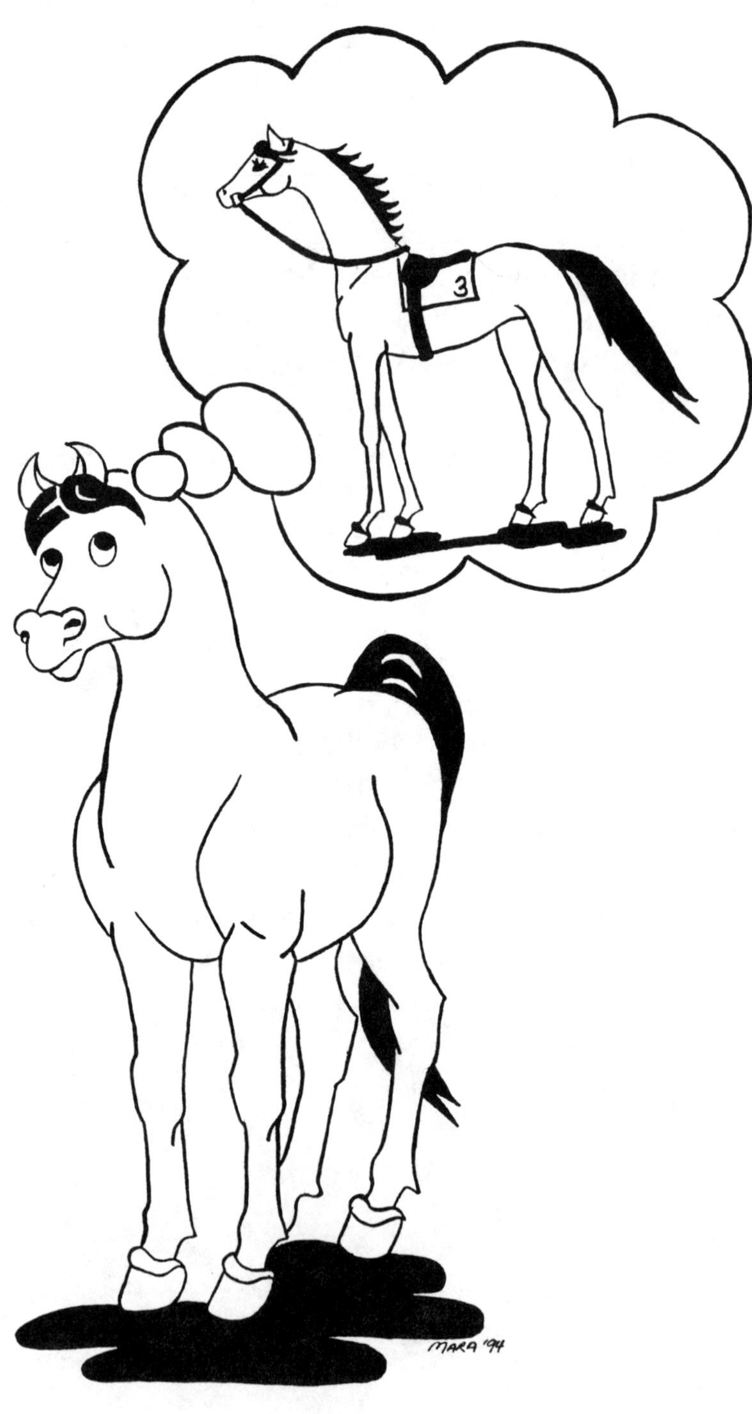
3
MARA '94

Second, more than likely, none of us are intended to be the size of a high-fashion runway model. A dear friend once told me, "You can't make a race horse out of draft horse stock." At the time, I thought, "Well, thanks one ***heck*** of a lot!" or something like that. But, she's right. We'll talk more about genetics under causation, but for now, start accepting this as reality.

That doesn't mean you have to be fat or unhealthy. It means you can achieve the best that you possibly can based on your own personal genetic make-up. A draft horse can't work if it is covered with blubber and out of shape. It needs to be as fit and trim as it can be. That won't make it look like a thoroughbred, just a *healthy* draft horse. If you're still not convinced, go back and re-read this chapter and think about your diet history. Have you been losing and gaining forever? Have you ever maintained a weight loss for any significant length of time after ending a deprivation diet? I doubt it. I'm right, am I not?

A journey of a thousand miles
must begin with
a single step.

- Lao-tzu

You can't diet forever and you can't maintain quick weight loss for any length of time if you don't diet forever—so here goes. You ready? You have a problem you want fixed? You want to take control? You bet! Let's look at causation (briefly—don't dwell on it) and a quick overview of what "cures" have been offered in the past in *Part Two*, then we'll move on to the *Nuts and Bolts* section of *Lifestyle Sculpting* in *Part Three*.

Don't skip *Part Two*. I want you to be reminded of all those goofy things you tried in your past that didn't work. It will help you stay on track with *Lifestyle Sculpting* to remember the quick weight-loss space suits, liquid fasts of milk shakes, and rice-only diets that you nearly killed yourself with over the years. Fad treatments don't work. *Lifestyle Sculpting* does. A major step in successful Sculpting is accepting and understanding causation so that you can release it and move forward. So dive into *Part Two* and get ready for *Part Three*. I'll see you there!

The thing always happens that you really believe in; and the belief in a thing makes it happen.

- Frank Lloyd Wright

PART TWO

Causation and "Cures"

Can You Really Cure Obesity?

The mind sins, not the body; if
there is no intention,
there is no blame.

- Titus Livius

One unable to dance blames the
unevenness of the floor.

- Malay Proverb

CHAPTER FOUR

Why Am I Fat?

People are always blaming their circumstances for what they are. I don't believe in circumstances. The people who succeed in this world are the people who get up and look for the circumstances they want, and if they can't find them, they make them.

- George Bernard Shaw

Two things that humans are best at are gossip and blame. Hanging over the back fence isn't our concern here, so let's look at causation and blame. Used for you, causation can be a tool. Used as a crutch, it can cripple. Causation is useful as long as you use it to say, "Okay, that's why I eat." or "Okay, that's why I'm built like a draft horse." From then on, the choice is yours. *Lifestyle Sculpting* is here to offer you options from which you can make educated choices. First, let's look at some commonly accepted causes of overweight which generally fall into one of three categories: genetic, physiological, or psychological.

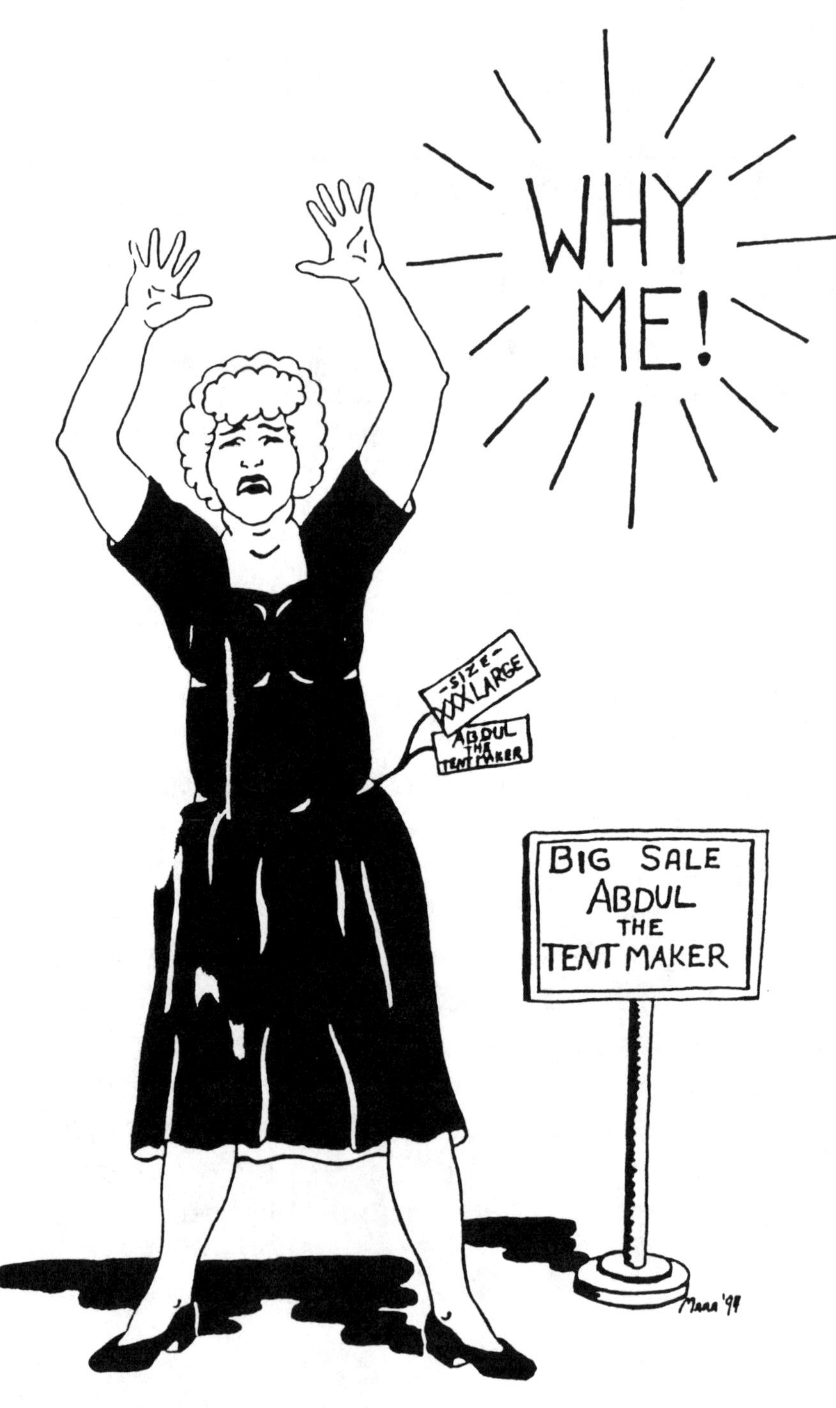
WHY ME!
-SIZE-
XXX LARGE
ABDUL THE TENT MAKER
BIG SALE
ABDUL
THE
TENT MAKER
Mara '94

First and foremost, *genetics*. No, you *can't* make a race horse out of draft horse stock. That's true enough. But, as I said, even draft horses can be fit and healthy. They have to be. They can't work efficiently, covered with blubber. So that excuse is out the window. You may have to work a little harder, eat a little less, or make more lifestyle changes than a genetic race horse, but if you get as fit and healthy as you can, who cares? You must also accept that you are the best you can be and be proud of that. So what if your shape is different from the runway models?

I have yet to hear my husband or other male members of my family say how attractive and sexy runway models are. The men I know say they like women with some curves and femininity. So accept the way you look, make your body the best it can be and revel in it. You'll feel great because you will have achieved a personal best and you will be better today than yesterday.

Just a side note on the genetics issue—keep in mind that you are fighting the "Survival of the Fittest" theory. Being able to store fat efficiently is what kept your ancient ancestors alive. The people who could maintain their body weight in

We are not permitted to choose
the frame of our destiny.
But what we put into it
is ours.

- Dag Hammarskjold

a famine survived, and that's why your ancestors lived to produce you. So accept the genetic power of your body; be glad of it, and get to work making it the best it can be. Always remember to go for your own personal best. *It doesn't matter what anyone else does.* Set a new personal best. You'll love it!

Physiological problems can certainly cause overweight. These are generally as simple as food allergies which can cause water retention or the hyperinsulinemia we discussed in *Chapter Two*. If you suspect hyperinsulinemia or food allergies, take a look in the recommended reading appendix. Two excellent books are reviewed there that deal with these issues. Always keep in mind that it is extremely rare for a person to have a thyroid problem or a true physiological binge eating disorder, but it does happen. You want to keep this in mind if you work hard at *Lifestyle Sculpting* and just **cannot** do it. There are reasons why you might have problems with the program, and we'll discuss those in reality checks and *Truth or Consequences*, but if you cannot put your finger on a food or emotional trigger, keep physiological eating disorders in mind to discuss with your physician. The most important thing to know about physiological problems is not to let them get

Many people today don't want
honest answers insofar as
honest means unpleasant
or disturbing.
They want a soft answer that
turneth away anxiety.

- Louis Kronenberger

you down. When you become aware of these influences, you can generally avoid or control them as you wish. Education is the key to control.

Psychological factors also draw fire in the debate of blame. These can include your personality traits, emotions, or psychological conditioning. A common place to point a finger that falls into this psychological spectrum is poor ol' mom. Yes, she may have helped turn you into a compulsive eater by feeding you every time you fell down, failed a class, or got dumped by a boy or girl—*but*, she didn't do it on purpose. She was trying to help. She was reverting to what *she* had learned from her mother and her community. How many of us grew up where a gathering was not a gathering without food and lots of it? A party, a funeral, an open house? Have you ever been to one, at least in the Midwest, without food? You name it, the food was there. My mother always cooked enough to feed an army, because God forbid we should run out of food and someone might ask for seconds or thirds. I do the same thing, as if my guests would die of starvation if I couldn't offer them more food!

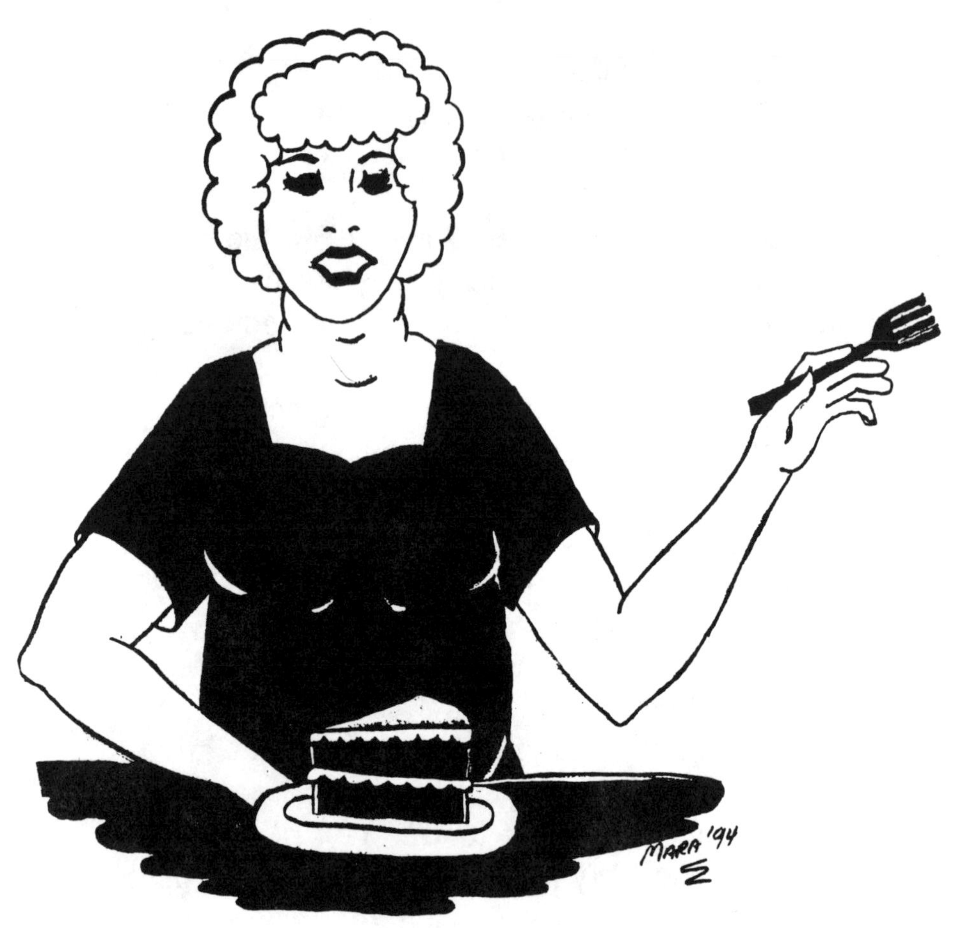

I'm fat because of genetics--and my mother raised me wrong--and TV is such a bad influence--and I have to cook for the family--and I work--and I don't have enough time to exercise...

Even knowing better as I do, the first thing I did when my granddaughter took her first fall from a horse was to offer her an ice cream cone when we finished the ride. The point is, what mom did (and dad, too), she did from love and concern and custom rather than to deliberately sabotage you. Now, it is up to you. Mom isn't standing there shoving that triple decker, chocolate fudge cake in your face now, is she? *You* are. Forgive mom and anyone else who fed you and take responsibility for yourself. You *choose* what to eat today—***you*** and you alone.

Along with psychological factors, we need to address personality traits. Many compulsive eaters are people pleasers, people who seek acceptance from others and who try to nurture *everyone*. My archaeology crew used to call me "mom" when I'd remind them of things they needed to take to the field or told them to be sure they had their rain gear, lunches, or water with them.

In my research, I found an extremely high percentage of overweight females who told people what they thought the person *wanted* to hear rather than what they actually thought. Also, many of us

Here's A Hint

Having a dinner party or house guests? Nobody needs a mountain of food nor do they need high fat foods. I have yet to hear of a recommendation of a high fat diet unless it is for some extreme medical condition. So do yourself and your guests a favor. Choose healthy, low fat foods and make plenty. If they want several servings, they are having a healthy entree'. Also choose foods that store in the refrigerator or freezer. That way, if not all the food is used, you can store it in one-portion servings and use it later. You will still be eating your healthier, low fat choices. To keep everyone from stuffing on the main entree', provide a fresh fruit and vegetable plate with low fat or fat free dressings for dipping before serving dinner. Be sure to have mineral water or club soda, fresh limes and lemons available to make a refreshing drink for those who do not want soda or alcohol before their meal. Simply pour mineral water over ice and add a lemon or lime twist.

For dessert, if you haven't fed them fruit on the appetizer tray, serve fresh fruit such as strawberries, bananas, or pineapple with dip made from low fat cream cheese which has been blended with fat free milk or creamer. Tastes sinful but has few fat grams!

are perfectionists. That's right, I said perfectionists. For years, if I couldn't look like Bo Derek (remember that "Perfect 10" body?), I was not even going to *try*. Why bother if I couldn't have a perfect body? Some of us have low self esteem and lack confidence. If we're overweight, chances are good we won't have to deal with being attractive to the opposite sex. For adolescents, being fat probably means they won't have to participate in sports and possibly fail because they won't be asked to play in the first place. How many of us are hiding behind our layers of social insulation?

In addition to genetics, physiology, and psychology, *time* and *convenience* take the rap too. You're too busy to cook, you *have* to eat fast food, the kids like it, your husband likes it—*whatever*. Well horsefeathers! There are more and more healthy choices to be had these days in fast food restaurants. (We'll look at those later in the *Nuts and Bolts section*.) You can make your own choices while the kids eat the high fat stuff. Remember though, you are doing them no favors by feeding them that junk either. A child fed high fat foods as an adolescent is more likely to be a fat

One doesn't discover new lands
without consenting to lose
sight of the shore
for a very long time.

- Andre' Gide

adult. If you do want to let them have fast foods as an occasional treat, then use the STOP Plan for yourself and think over your choices and the consequences. If *you* want fast food too, fine. When our business was burglarized recently, nothing short of a double-bacon cheeseburger, large fries, and a Classic Coke would do. The point is—**think**. Then, if you want the high fat food, ***choose*** it, but if you really don't, then make a healthy choice instead. It is up to you.

Take time to sift through your history. What are your personality traits? How about your genetic background? What did your mother and father and grandparents look like? Have I hit a few chords here? Once you have figured out what you believe has caused your overweight, remember that causation is just that—it lets you define what factors started your problem and which ones have lead to your tendency to overeat, ***but*** today's problem is the pounds hanging on your body *now*—not what happened twenty years ago or how busy you are today or that milk that makes you put on five pounds overnight because you're allergic to it. **You** put those pounds there by making the choices you did.

Those who cannot remember the past
are condemned to repeat it.

- George Santayana

Accept the causes for your overweight problem and then file them in an imaginary garbage can where they belong. The solution to the problem lies not in its causation but in assuming responsibility. The responsibility is yours and yours alone. *Lifestyle Sculpting* is here to teach you how to accept that truth and to take control of your eating problems. **Now!**

Here's A Hint

It seems to be human nature to seek "quick fixes." You will see in the text there aren't any quick fixes to be found. As you can tell from the *Author Photo* on the back of this book, I am an avid horsewoman. My husband and I constantly have clients who want a fully trained show horse, safe to ride and drive in the ring and out on trails in 30 to 90 days. (We call these "ninety-day wonders"!) Well, guess what?--won't happen, can't be done. Now I better qualify that *fast* before those of you who know horses get a pen in hand to write me a letter! Yes, we can make a horse do those things fairly quickly just as you can lose weight quickly with a reduction diet. Will the quick fix last any better on a horse's education than your weight loss will? No way! A horse has to go through kindergarten, elementary school, high school, and college. Depending on what you want to do, he may even need post graduate work and ad hoc research! This process takes **years.** So why do we always want things done yesterday? I honestly don't know and can't answer that. With the horses, it is sometimes money. Training for that length of time is expensive. Most of the time I think it is just our hurry-up-and-get-it-without-working-for-it attitude. I think our weight loss is the same. We have suffered pain, humiliation, and discrimination. We have faced all the problems overweight brings. We want it over with--*yesterday*. Sorry folks, that isn't going to happen. Just like the development of a world class horse, these things take time. Don't rush yourself. In the end, the wait will be worth it, *more* than worth it. You will know that the end result will **last**. You will not need to fear the return of your hated overweight. ***Take your time, don't hurry.*** Take one level at a time, going to the next level only when you are fully prepared. It will be worth the wait!

CHAPTER FIVE

Are There Cures For Obesity?

You gain strength, courage and confidence by every experience in which you really stop and look fear in the face. You are able to say to yourself, "If I lived through this horror, I can take the next thing that comes along." You must do something you think you cannot do.

- Eleanor Roosevelt

Here we hit more good news/bad news. *Is there a cure for obesity?* **No.** Obesity is a symptom of another problem. You don't *cure* symptoms, you *treat* them. To "fix" obesity permanently, you must cure its cause. So I ask again, can you cure obesity? No! *Is there a way to fix the lifestyle that brought it on?* **You bet!** *Do all the diets and "cures" floating around out there work?* **Not a chance.** Think about it. If even *one* of them worked well, do you think people would still be designing, selling, and trying different diets? Of course not. The one diet book that worked would rule the diet industry.

Here's A Hint

Let's play a word association game. Get a pen and paper. Ready? Good. Now write down every word that pops into your head when you think of a diet.

Done? How many of those words have a positive connotation? Pretty bad, aren't they? Negative images leap into your consciousness whenever you consider a diet. Do you really want to try another one? Do you want to place your future health and well-being in the hands of another diet guru? I don't think so. Get busy reading and leave those blasted diets alone. Every time you are tempted to try a quick fix diet, grab a pen and do this exercise again. Do it as often as necessary to keep yourself from leaping back onto that diet carousel. You can do it! Resist the urge and get busy *Lifestyle Sculpting* instead.

Diets—we've all been on them, tried anything and everything to lose weight and keep it off.

The number of diets out there is infinite—rice only, carbohydrates only, high carb, low carb, high protein, low protein, low fat... I could go on and on. You name it and it's been tried (mostly by *me*!). I have a bookshelf (or two or three) full of nothing but diet books. Some I bought for research; most I have tried at one time or another during my yo-yoing years. Some of them actually have good information that will be mentioned in the *Recommended Reading Appendix*. Most I found to be useless, representing (or misrepresenting) quick fixes for lifelong problems. The solutions presented in many diets are not solutions at all. They entail regimens of food or exercise you can't possibly live with for a lifetime, whether it's because you are not physically up to it or because you simply do not like them, and thus won't stick with them.

Drugs? We know there are all kinds out there—over the counter, prescription, natural, holistic, herbs. Does any of it really work alone, without a strict, reduced calorie diet and increased exercise? No way. And while they are busy

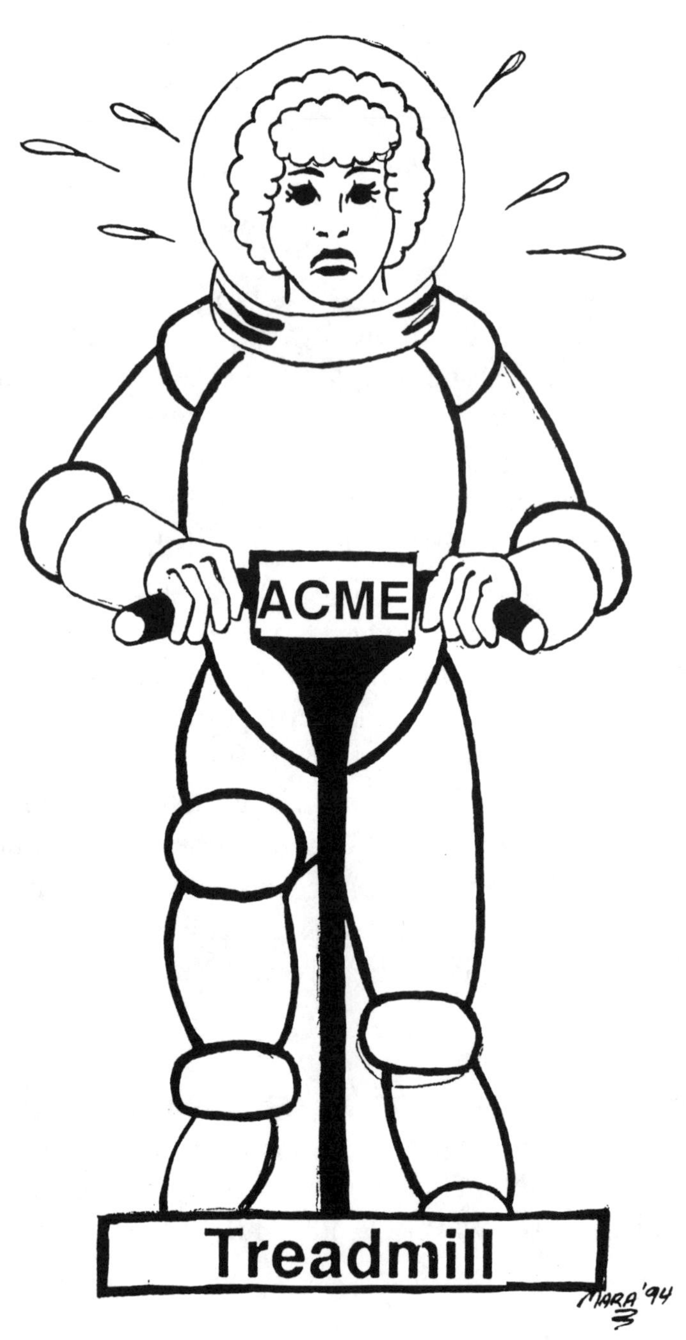
ACME
Treadmill
MARA '94

doing nothing except draining your bank account, many drugs can be harming your health. The key to whether to use drugs to lose weight is simple. *Can you take this medication forever?* If not, what's the point? Use your common sense. I know you have it; we all do. It is obvious that as soon as you quit taking weight loss drugs or appetite suppressants, the weight will come back on, oftentimes more than you had lost to start with. Many of these drugs cause serious side effects and can be addictive. If you can't stop taking it without your body reacting to its withdrawal, do you really want it in your system?

Then, we see the gimmicks—machines for thin thighs, hundreds of new aerobics tapes, sweating off pounds of fat wearing a space suit on a treadmill, step aerobics, weight lifting. I don't know about you, but I have a zillion of these. Do I use them? Hardly ever (some of my favorites will be mentioned in the *Recommended Tapes Appendix*).

When I designed *Lifestyle Sculpting*, if I couldn't do an exercise or sport on a horse, it didn't get done. To me sports meant horses, exercise meant

Here's A Hint

One major premise of *Lifestyle Sculpting* is to not deprive yourself of foods you love. Cut down on them or make them in low fat ways, but **do not** forbid yourself to ever enjoy them. This is a recipe of a family favorite that my mother used to make. I refused to give it up for reasons that went beyond taste. Yes, I enjoy this dish but it was also something of my mother's. It has a special place in my recipe file and my heart. It is one of my comfort foods. So try it and I hope you enjoy it. If it doesn't appeal, try a favorite of your own in a smaller size or low fat version.

PINEAPPLE SALAD

1 can sliced pineapple packed in juice
1 T flour
2 T sugar or use substitute to equal this
2 eggs
Cottage cheese, low fat or fat free

Drain pineapple and place juice in pan. Blend in flour, sugar and eggs. Cook over low heat, stirring constantly until it thickens. This will happen quickly so watch it closely when it starts to thicken and remove immediately from heat. This takes only a few minutes. Chill.

Place lettuce leaves on a plate. Add two pineapple slices. Spoon on low fat or fat free cottage cheese. Pour pineapple sauce over cottage cheese. Sprinkle with paprika for color.

Makes four substantial servings or six moderate ones.

horses, ***fun*** meant horses. That's all there was to it. I wasn't going to jog, walk, or do aerobics. Oh, I tried. Two days and I was bored silly. Not to mention that I am a total klutz and had a terrible time keeping up with the majority of beginner aerobics tapes. Yes, I have increased my activities, and I even walk on a treadmill now because I learned how to do it at a time of day and in a manner I enjoyed (more on that later). These changes came about gradually though. I didn't leap off the couch at 265 pounds and start pumping iron! The point is, most of these spot reducing gadgets and exercise tapes are just a waste of hard-earned money. Either you won't use them routinely or they simply don't work.

While this may all seem like a passel of bad news, it isn't! The good news is you *can* and *will* lose weight permanently without ever going on another diet or exercise regimen again. You don't need to spend another dollar on gimmicks or useless and damaging drugs.

You can't make huge lifestyle changes all at once and expect them to stick. Don't try to trim calories, banning favorite foods while adding

As for the future, your task is not to foresee, but to enable it.

- Antoine de Saint-Exupery

rigorous exercises you hate all at once. How long do you think that will last? For me, it always lasted two or three days, if that. The older I got, the shorter the length of time I stuck to that stuff. I believe I was realizing it just didn't work and wasn't worth the effort before it finally sank into my brain. Don't do this to yourself. Accept the truth. Weight loss occurs and is maintained *permanently* through *Lifestyle Sculpting*.

Face it, you do have to make changes, **but** they are easy, enjoyable, small steps. Don't leap into it all at once. You gained this weight over time and have probably carried it most of your life. Don't expect to lose it overnight. *Do* expect to lose it with minor effort, making small changes, one or two at a time. If it takes several months or a year, so what! You will feel better each and every day as the weight comes off with seemingly little effort. When you hit a plateau, you will know the weight is not coming back because you didn't lose it with a diet; you lost it with *Lifestyle Sculpting*. As your eating habits improve gradually and you get your mind and body active, you will begin to feel marvelous. Count on it!

Whatever you can do or dream you can, begin it. Boldness has genius, power, and magic in it.

- W.H. Murray

It's time. Enough background. Move to *Part Three* and find out how to start, then get busy—TODAY! Don't wait another minute. Make one change today and others will follow. You'll never go back unless you choose to.

Here's A Hint

As you begin losing weight the temptation will be great to run out and buy smaller clothes. ***Don't Do It!*** Your current clothes will be getting looser and you'll feel *great.* You will feel small in those clothes that are a little loose around the waist or wherever. If you give in to the urge and go buy a size or two smaller, guess what? You will have a momentary feeling of elation to see yourself in those smaller clothes. You'll look smaller. And then, reality will hit. Those clothes will feel tight and too small. The first time you wash that newer size pair of jeans, you'll be dancing in them to get the zipper closed. How will you feel? **FAT!!** What will you do? **EAT!!**

Don't do this. Wear the clothes you have now until they are darned near falling off, then go buy the next smaller size (not two or three sizes smaller!) and wear those relatively loose clothes until they feel like *they're* falling off. Then do it again. It will be worth the patience and extra money for in-between sizes if you feel good and stay with your plan.

PART THREE

Lifestyle Sculpting

Nuts and Bolts

Procrastination is the fear
of success. People procrastinate
because they are afraid
of the success that they know
will result if they move
ahead now. Because success
is heavy and carries
responsibility with it,
it is much easier to
procrastinate and live on the
"someday I'll" philosophy.

- Dennis Waitley

CHAPTER SIX

Getting Started Today!

Failure is impossible.
- Susan B. Anthony

There is no such thing as failure.
- Kathleen Wells

"Failure is impossible." That is so important, I am repeating it. I would like to be presumptuous enough to add to it as well—*failure* is impossible because there *is* no such thing. Failure implies that a new thing was tried and a failure occurred. *Not possible*. If something new was tried and it didn't work, the person learned a valuable lesson. One thing you learn in scientific research is that it is just as important to find out what doesn't work (null-hypothesis) as finding out what *does* (hypothesis). Education is never a failure—never. If you try a diet and lose weight, then stop the diet and gain the weight back, have you failed? I say a resounding *NO*! You learned about yourself and about that diet you tried. I can't say it enough

Never give in.
Never. Never. Never. Never.

- Winston Churchill

nor emphasize it too strongly. You *learned* something and education of any kind is never, never a waste nor a failure. So, take all that experience and education about dieting that you have picked up over the years and say, "*No more!*" They say, "Never say never," but in this case, go ahead! Make yourself a promise that you will NEVER diet again.

Believe me, diets can be tempting. As you are working the Lifestyle Sculpting Program, a new diet or pill will come along and your fingers will be itching to buy the book or the pill. Maybe, you think to yourself, if I just try this one for a week or two to make my weight come off faster, then I can go back to *Lifestyle Sculpting*. I know I never fail to stop and look at these myself, picking up the book or magazine in the grocery line that has a headline about quick weight loss. Don't give in. It won't work; it isn't worth it. And you can sabotage all the good changes you have made with *Lifestyle Sculpting*. *Stick to your plan.* Remember, *it doesn't matter how long it takes to lose, as long as you are getting more healthy and happy every day.* Tell yourself this a thousand times a day if you need to, until you believe it.

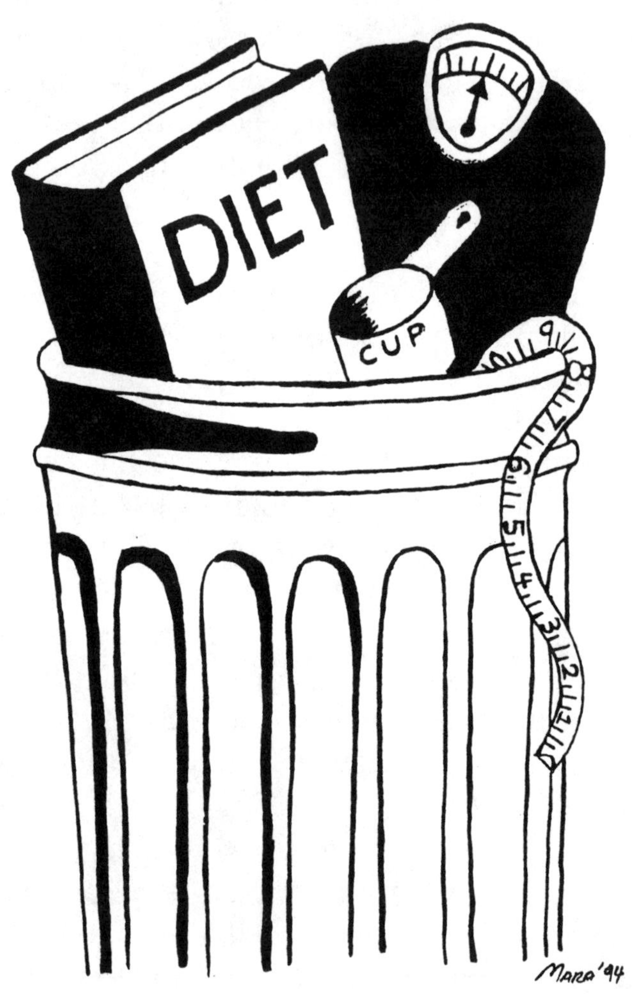
DIET
CUP
MARA '94

So, *let's get to it*! There are some things you need to do to get ready. We've already said more than enough about banning diets, drugs, and gimmicks. I want you to add to that list your measuring spoons, food scales, bathroom scales, tape measures, and dress sizes. Throw them out, hide them in a deep, dark closet—but stay away from them! All of these measures are a means to continue an obsession with weight loss. How much you lose doesn't matter. What dress size or pants size you wear doesn't matter. It is physiologically impossible for you *not* to lose weight if you more often than not make healthy, lower calorie, lower fat food choices while increasing your activities and maintaining a good attitude about yourself. You *will* lose weight—no ifs, ands, or buts about it.

I recently watched a weight loss infomercial, where the participants were saying the plan founder wouldn't let them measure how much weight they lost. Instead, they kept track of how many dress sizes they lost. I say, "Same, same." You are *still* measuring and being obsessed with the loss itself. This is not where you want your focus to be. Personally, my heart says to throw

*Do not set your eyes on
things far off.*

- Pythian Odes

out the scales and measuring tapes, but the tightwad portion of my brain says to stick them in a closet where it is difficult to get to them.

Also, as I will discuss later, there is one place and time, and only one, where these items might come in handy as a reality check. For now though, to get started, bury them, hide them, forget you own them so that you will not be tempted to use them.

Lifestyle Sculpting is not about keeping score or seeing how fast you can reduce. It is about changes. Your tastes in foods will change; your body will change; your energy level will change; your interests will broaden. That's what we're after. Losing weight is a by-product of those changes, so forget about keeping track and get on with it.

I would like to say something here about before and after pictures. You'll notice an evident lack of "after" pictures in this book. My "before" picture is here to show you where I was when I designed the *Lifestyle Sculpting* and STOP programs. The "Author's Photo" was taken when I had lost my first forty-five pounds but was still well above my healthy weight. "Before" pictures are helpful if you use them as a reminder. It's kind of like a

We (Americans) suffer primarily not from our vices or our weaknesses, but from our illusions. We are haunted, not by reality, but by those images we have put in place of reality.

- Daniel Boorstin

picture of a dirty, grungy city. You can look at it and say, "I've been there and I'm never going back." "After" pictures are most often illusions, non-reality. If you take a picture the day you hit your goal weight (another fallacy), what happens if nature says that your weight is too light for you and you come back up ten pounds before stabilizing? You'll throw up your hands, say what good is it all anyway, and start overeating. Your "after" picture should be visible to you only when you look in the mirror—*the way you look today*. No matter what your weight is, and we all fluctuate somewhat, you are better today than yesterday if you are *Lifestyle Sculpting*. Be happy with that and don't hold up some fantasy picture to try to live up to.

So called motivational pictures of skinny, beautiful models cut out of magazines go right out with "after" pictures for the same reason. Look at your "before" picture to remember that you don't want to ever visit *that* place again (as if you could ever forget the years of humiliation and pain!), then pat yourself on the back for a job well done ***today*** and for being as healthy as you can be ***today***.

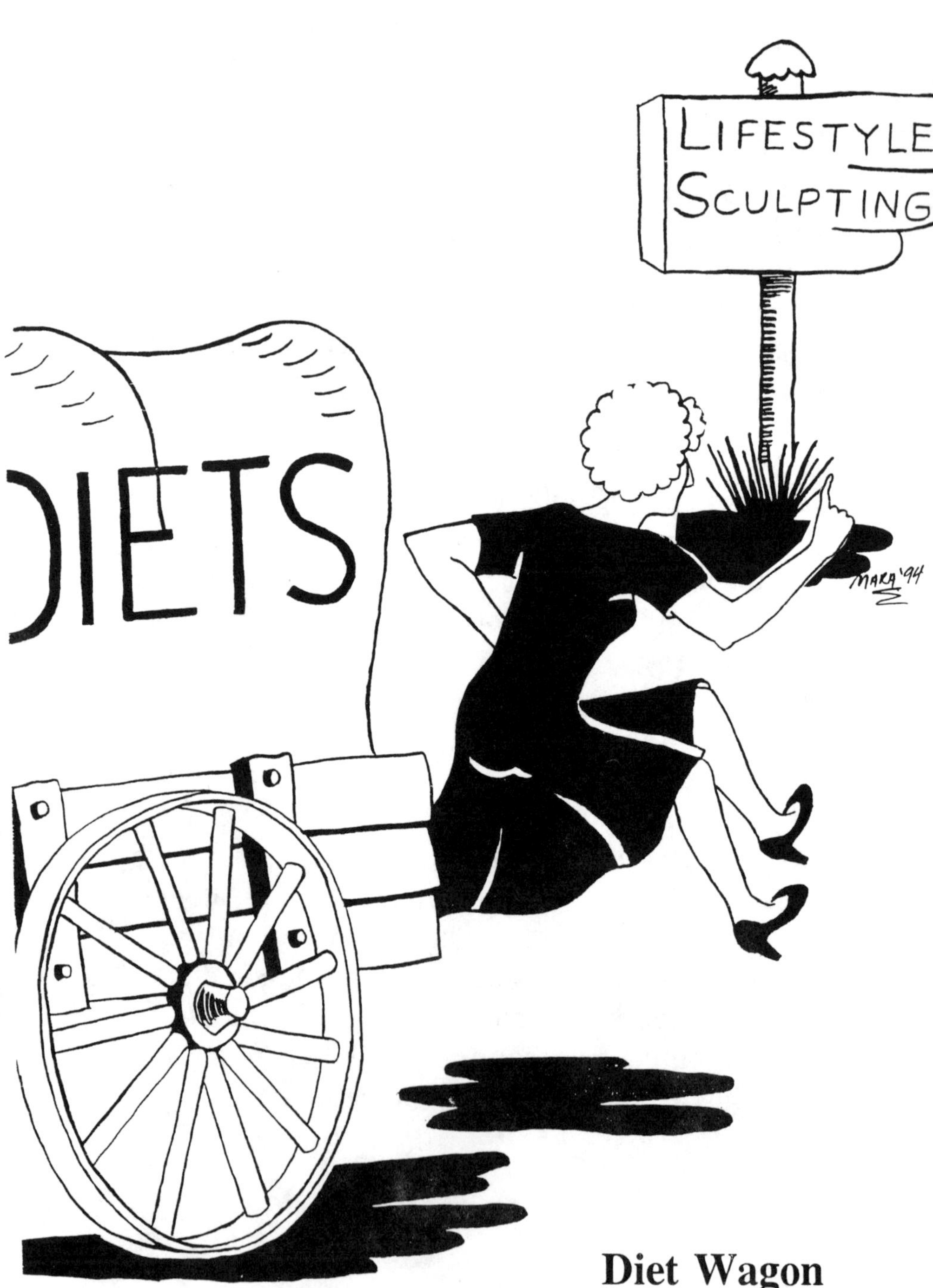

Diet Wagon

The bottom line reasoning for the success of Lifestyle Sculpting is so simple, it's scary. You'll read this and go, "Why on earth didn't I think of this? What took so long?" We've already decided that diets won't keep your weight off—take it off, yes, keep it off, no. It follows that if you lose weight by dieting while you are supposedly learning lifestyle habits and eating habits that are better, that won't work either.

Wait a minute, you say? Semantics? No, it's not. Think about it. Have you ever lost weight *because* of a lifestyle change? Have you gone from one high fat, high calorie food to another lower in fat and calories and lost a few pounds? Have you done reduced calorie diets and lost weight while you tried to learn what you needed to eat when the weight was off? That's backwards!

Make a change. I'll teach you how. And then you'll lose weight as a result of that change—not because of a diet or exercise but because of that change! Diets mean deprivation, drastic measures, constant weighing, portion control, and a wagon you can fall off of. *Lifestyle Sculpting* means

Here's A Hint

When you go out, avoid the eat-all-you-want meals. It is too tempting to want to get your money's worth. You will be tempted to force down just a little more, even if you're stuffed, because it's "free."

Also watch out for all-you-can-eat salad bars. Only frequent these if you can turn down the potato salad and pasta salad made with oils and the high fat dressings. If you can stick to the fruits and vegetables with low fat dressing and to the nice dinner rolls without butter, go for it.

Otherwise, order a dinner salad and a regular meal. A salad bar is not a weight loss tool unless you control *it* rather than it controlling *you*!

simple changes. Simple changes, *that's all.* Changing from one food to another, one at a time, or changing from watching an art class on television to going out and taking one at the local community center. So throw all those diets, drugs, and gimmicks out and let's start Sculpting! It worked for me. It will work for you.

This Is Me!

Well, here it is—the infamous "before" picture! Here are just two of the many that I have from the years and years of yo-yoing that I have done all my life.

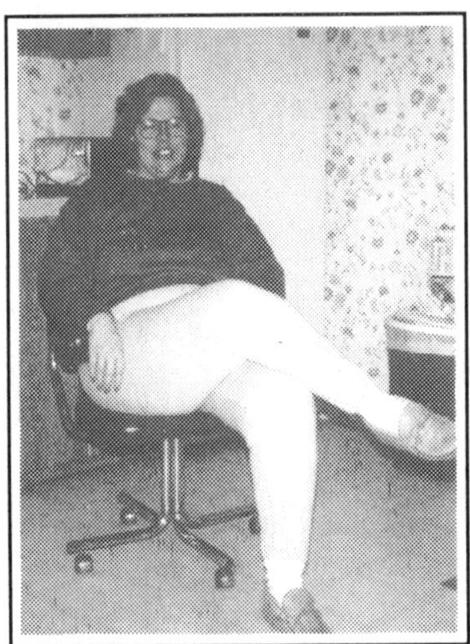

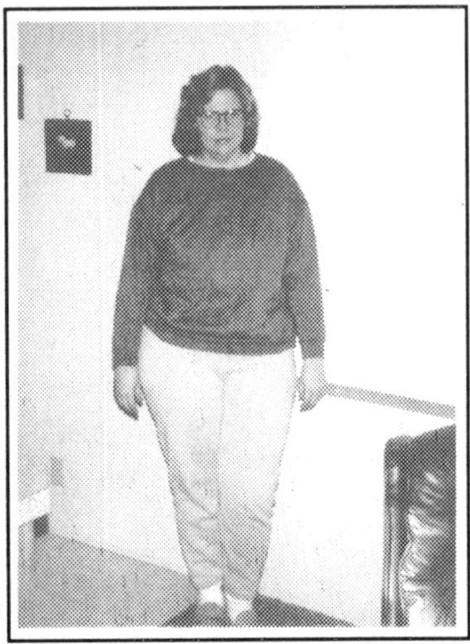

Born at almost eleven pounds (that's right, eleven), I started out in this life fat. My weight went up and down for the first forty years of my life. In the early years, it rose and fell according to my growth spurts and whether or not I had a horse to ride through my teen years. Do you older folks remember the tuna commercials with Minnie the Whale? That's what kids called me when I was in elementary school. Several times, I ran home from the local pool in tears after being teased because I had dared to wear a bathing suit in public. During the brief periods when I would lose that "baby" fat and slim down, I felt great. Before long though, the fat would return and my self-esteem would go into a tailspin.

During my adult years, the weight came and went with crises—from the loss of my mother when I was twenty-one to a divorce to the stress of starting college as a non-traditional student at the age of thirty-two. After graduation, I once again began to lose weight when I became an archaelogist for the U.S. Forest Service. Hiking in the mountains helped with the weight loss until a minor heart problem developed and I suddenly became sedentary. The weight came back on in record time and topped out at 265 pounds, my highest *ever*. Sick and tired, *literally*, of being overweight, I finally decided enough was enough. Nothing in the "real world" offered me diddly for permanent weight loss. Being the daughter of an engineer, I did the thing that always came naturally around our house—I got out a pencil and paper and set about solving the problem myself. The results of my brainstorming are the two programs that I used to lose weight myself—the programs now known as *Lifestyle Sculpting* and the STOP Plan that are the basis of this book.

I am excited about sharing these with you so that you too can know what permanent weight loss feels like and know the exhilaration of success. I'm here to tell you it feels *great!* This *"before"* picture is all the motivation I need, added to how good I feel for the first time in many years, to keep me using my programs.

I wish you all the same success and happiness. Believe me, if ***I*** could go from the way I was in this picture to what I am today—healthy, happy, and thinner—**YOU** can too!

The reason men oppose progress
is not that they hate
progress, but that they
love inertia.

- Elbert Hubbard

Most folks are as happy as they make up their minds to be.

- Abraham Lincoln

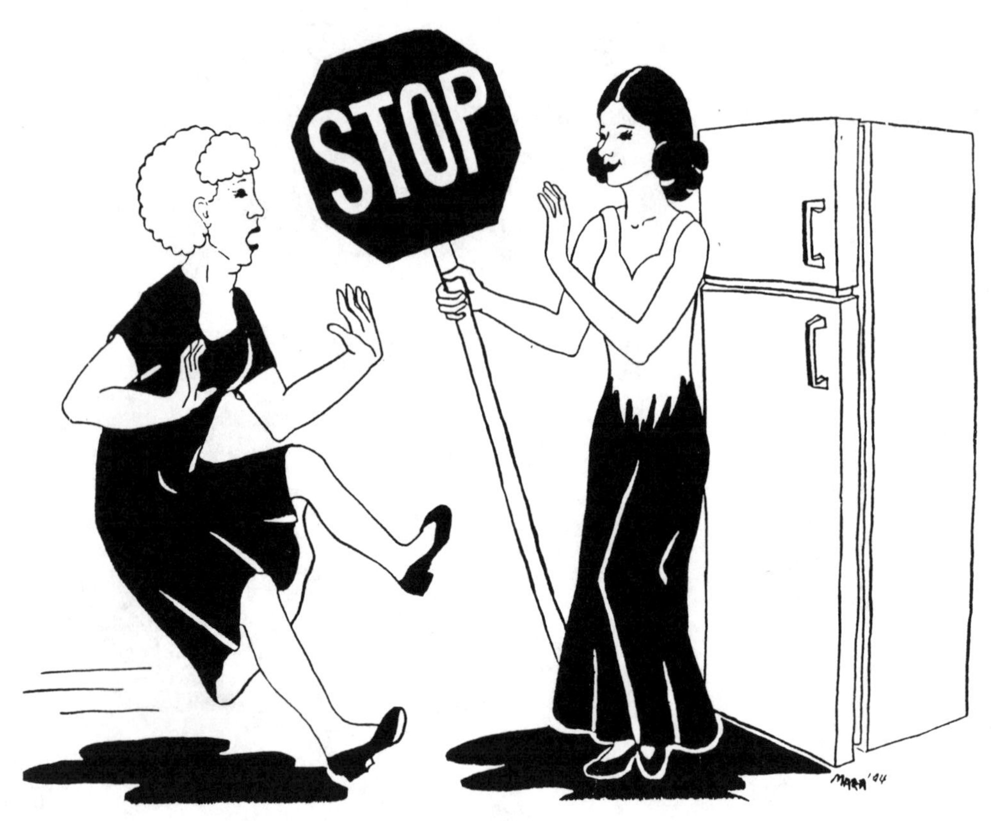

STOP Plan

S=Stop T=Think O=Options P=Proceed

CHAPTER SEVEN

STOP to Start

All glory comes from daring to begin.
- Eugene F. Ware

It's time to get serious. We've been discussing causation and background information long enough. The first phase to permanent weight loss is awareness. The STOP Plan will empower you by making you aware of what you are doing. Many compulsive eaters can eat all day (grazing) and not be able to tell you what they had, how it tasted, or if it was worth the calories.

I don't believe it's necessary to write down every morsel of food that passes through your lips, to keep endless food diaries, or to weigh and measure every bite you eat. Common sense and *moderation*, to use another good friend's favorite word, are the keys to weight loss. The STOP Plan is a tool for raising your level of awareness so that you can apply these other tools effortlessly.

The strongest principle of growth lies in human choice.

- George Eliot (pen name of Mary Ann Evans, 1819-1880)

STOP is an acrostic for the Stop Plan system. "S" simply stands for STOP! That means *now*—before you take that first bite. I'm not telling you to stop and not eat it. I am simply telling you to *STOP* and don't do a thing until you work the rest of the program. If you still want that bite, you can eat it then. The choice is always yours. You can wait a minute or two, can't you? So, STOP!—then continue with the plan.

"T" reminds you to "Think!" Make eating a *conscious* endeavor, not a mindless habit. *THINK!* Why do you want to eat? Are you really hungry or just angry, depressed, bored, or ______ (you can fill in your own blank)? It may just look good. We have hundreds of reasons for eating.

"O" offers "Options." We all have them. We all exercise them. We all make deliberate choices. Even no action at all is a choice. Your options are simple. If you are truly hungry, eat and don't feel guilty about it. If you are angry, depressed, or hurt, *express* your feelings—in a kind and mature way. Write in your journal, talk, yell, but do not eat if you can help it. Bored? Get off your butt

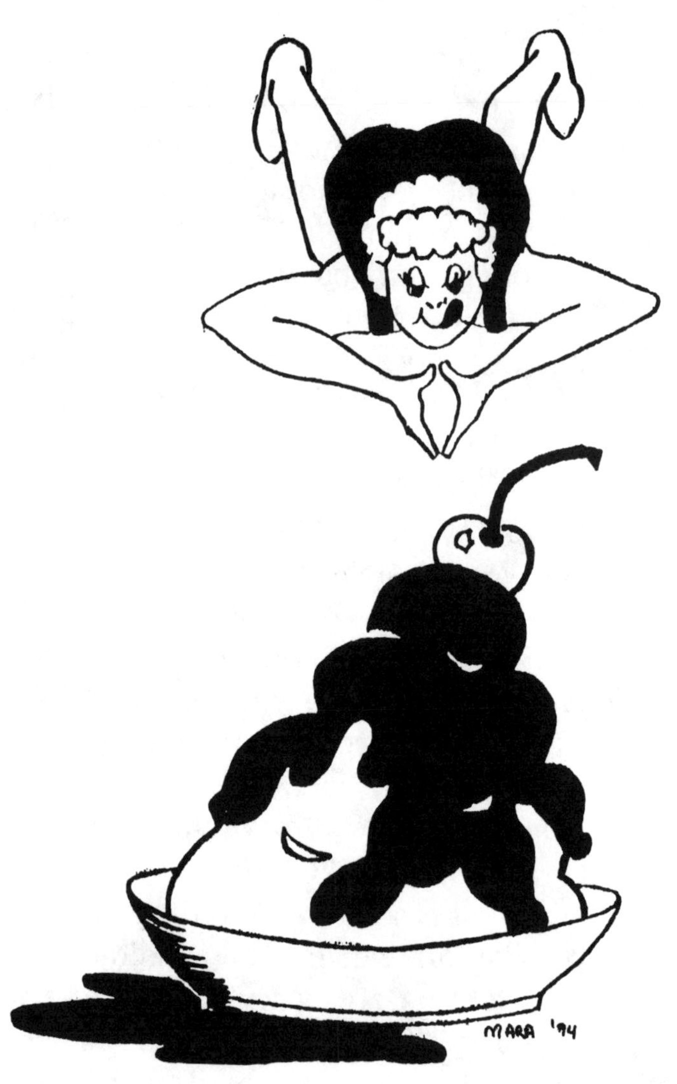

I thought about it. I want it.
I don't feel guilty about it.

and do something, *any*thing! Don't sit there and whine about having nothing to do. There are a multitude of experiences out that front door just waiting for you. The choice is yours.

"P" stands for "Proceed." *Go for it*! With caution, always. Pay attention to yourself, know your feelings, know when you are really hungry. Work at making the healthy, guilt-free choice for you. If the choice that is important to you is a hot fudge sundae and you have considered the options and the consequences, eat it. Don't feel guilty. It is *your* choice.

As you work the STOP Plan, become aware of your hunger, of the taste of the food you are eating. Break your old habits by using the STOP Plan. If you're eating because someone set a plate in front of you and you really don't want it, dump it. If you order something and it doesn't taste as good as you thought it would, dump it. I don't care about the Great Depression. It's over. I do care about starving children in other countries and here in the United States, but that plate of food you don't eat won't get to them anyway. Dump it. There's no law against it.

A straight path never leads anywhere except to the objective.

- Andre' Gide

Don't reach for food without thinking first. If you're having a bad day, work the plan. If you go through the steps and your options and realize you are in dire need of hot apple pie a' la mode and nothing less will do, then accept that your weight loss might be delayed a few days by the extra calories and fat and dive in. The choices are yours. The consequences are yours. Is the comfort food really more important to you on that day than the weight loss? If so, *go for it!* Don't feel guilty about it. Don't regret it. You deserve to have what you truly *need.* If something else will fill the place of the comfort food, and you will find that to be the case more often than not, then go with that instead of the food. Otherwise, do a swan dive, face down, into that melting ice cream and apple pie. Eat it slowly. Taste it. Enjoy it. Savor it. Make every calorie and fat gram count. Then get back to your program.

The STOP Plan is for anyone who needs to lose weight from Normal Overweights to Binge Eaters. Simply by making yourself aware of when, why, and what you eat, you can slow down your ingestion of food. Any calories saved from one day or meal to another will lead to weight loss.

Here's A Hint

Are you a two sandwich person? I sure was. And on many days, I still am. Try this: take your favorite bread (most are low or fat free just by nature) and spread a thin layer of low fat or fat free mayonnaise on it. Use Dijon mustard if you want fat free, spicy flavor. Split a small can of white meat chicken in half and place that on the bread. Pile on (Dagwood-style!) lettuce, tomato, onion, sprouts, whatever veggies you want. Then *dig in*! Still hungry when you finish that one? Do it again. It was low in fat but nutritious and delicious—so enjoy! If you haven't tried it yet, get some pita bread and put the chicken in the bottom. Add a little low fat mayo or mustard, stuff with veggies and eat!

As your tastes and needs change and are satisfied in different ways, you will make more changes and lose more weight naturally through *Lifestyle Sculpting*. And the weight loss will last because you haven't dieted, drugged, or fasted the pounds away. Remember, you can't fall off the diet carousel if you don't climb on board in the first place.

The STOP Plan can help define those of you with true physiological eating disorders. Work the plan meticulously. Do your best to become aware of when and why you are eating. If you are unable to stop binging or if your eating continues for hours in spite of working the STOP Plan, then seek some help from a qualified physician. Be prepared to tell the physician what you have tried, how much you are eating, when, and why (if you know). There's hope and help out there for you. New solutions for these eating disorders are on the horizon.

Awareness. That's Phase One. So get busy and start implementing the STOP Plan today. You will begin losing weight simply by becoming aware of your grazing so that you are conscious of what you

*You can change anything you want,
but you can't change everything
you want.*

- John-Roger & Peter McWilliams

are eating. You will begin turning junk food down more often than not. You will begin turning large portions down and opting for smaller "samples" of high fat, high calorie foods. You will do this *if* you work the STOP Plan and *think* before you eat.

When you do this, you will begin to lose weight. Now that you are tuned into your eating and are aware of when you are eating and why, it's time to start *Lifestyle Sculpting*.

It is better to begin in the evening than not at all.

- English Proverb

The great thing in this world
is not so much where we are, but
in what direction we are moving.

- Oliver Wendell Holmes

CHAPTER EIGHT

Lifestyle Sculpting
Food Changes First

The best and most beautiful things in the world cannot be seen or touched. They must be felt with the heart.
- Helen Keller

I chose this quote because I want you to begin to sense your own good health in your heart. The scale doesn't take this into account, the tape measure won't show it, and the smaller dress size won't reflect it. The importance of *Lifestyle Sculpting* is in the changes you can make in your health, both physical and psychological. You will feel the results of these changes within. With each better day, you will feel progress is being made. You'll have more energy, better self-esteem, and pride. You can do this yourself—no diets, no drugs, no gimmicks. With no more help than someone putting you on the right track, you can make the difference in your own life, starting today.

Nothing great was ever achieved without enthusiasm.

- Ralph Waldo Emerson

There are three areas of your life which need sculpting if you are to succeed in permanent weight loss. These are your eating habits, your activities, and stress management. You may be one of the lucky few Normal Overweights who doesn't need work in all of these areas. Most compulsive eaters, however, need some changes made in all three of these aspects of their daily lives.

The thing I want to stress here is that you must take *baby steps* in these areas. Don't sit down and set yourself out a list of impossible goals. I was famous for deciding to cut my calories to 1,000 (or less) a day, eliminating all of my favorite foods, and saying I would get up at 5 a.m. to work out before going to the office. Right! Did it work? Not a snowball's chance in hell! You can't make immense changes all at once and expect to succeed. You can make changes one level at a time and never miss the old you or the things you cut out. Each of these three subjects is of equal importance. Most of you will not maintain permanent weight loss without working in all three areas.

Here's A Hint

When you dine out, order the small serving first—the half salad, petite cut, whatever. Is it carved in granite that you only have one shot to order? That you can't place a second order if you want to? Of course not!! Order and eat the half chef salad or petite cut steak. If you are still hungry when you are done, then order something else—even if it's a salad to which you add fat free dressing. Most of the time, though, you will be full when you finish what you ordered. Think about it. How often do you finish a meal and push back from the table overfull, commenting that a half sandwich or small burger would have been plenty? Follow your instinct that a small serving is adequate, not your compulsive have-to-have-food-or-die instinct, and order *small*.

Before we go further into *Lifestyle Sculpting*, I want to remind you of the importance of checking with your physician. Yes, we all know we are overweight and need to lose. We don't need another person to tell us that. But you have been sedentary and overweight for quite some time in most cases. Don't make sudden changes without being sure you have no underlying medical problems. Discuss this plan with your physician and get her or his blessing. Getting approval for even gradual food changes is especially important if you have any medical concerns such as high cholesterol or diabetes. So be safe. See a physician first.

You might be surprised. Your doctor may actually try to talk you *out* of trying to lose weight until you explain the combination of changes the program calls for. My own internist told me not once, but several times, not to lose weight. In all of his years of experience he had never had a single patient with a permanent weight loss success story.

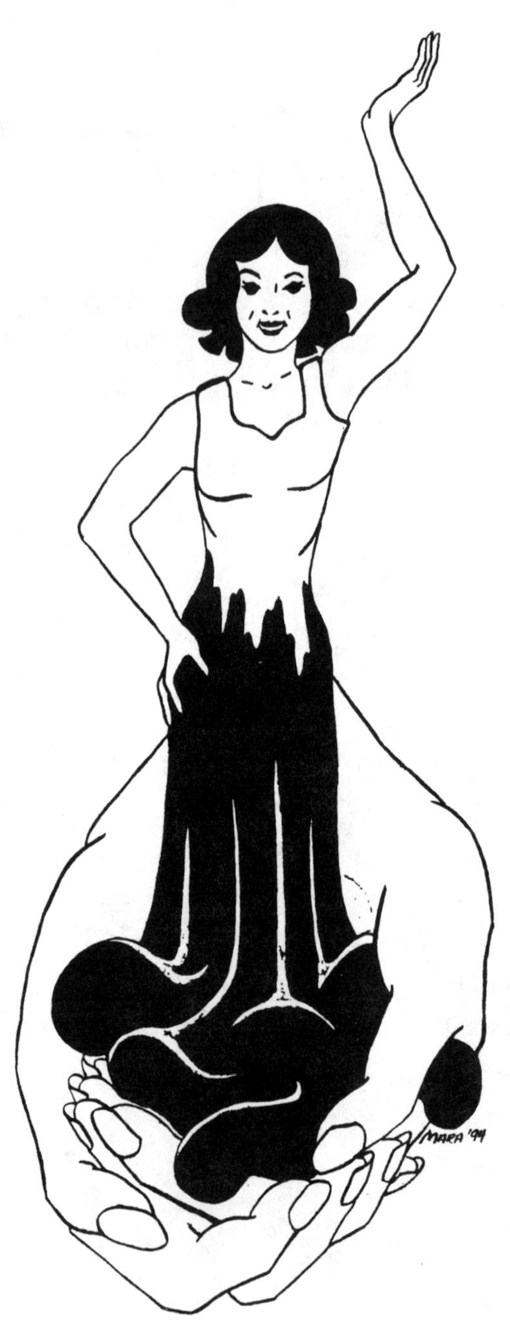
MARA '94

The dangers of yo-yoing are becoming well documented. Read this program, discuss it with your doctor and make a conscious decision to create change. *Mold your life like a lump of wet clay*. Peel off one layer after another until you have your masterpiece. You can make that pile of wet earth anything you *want* it to be.

The STOP Plan was the first part of the program and the actual *Lifestyle Sculpting*, the second. *Lifestyle Sculpting* is broken down into three phases with several easy steps in each phase. Food changes are probably the easiest part of *Lifestyle Sculpting*, so we'll start there. That may seem surprising to you, but what we eat is far less important to us than you may now realize.

Lifestyle sculpting of food choices happens in stages. At each point, you decide what you will change or give up and what you won't. If you have things you absolutely won't give up, then just cut down on them. My big one—roasted chicken or turkey skin. Can't you see it, crisp and brown? I can practically *smell* a roast chicken right now. It's the "s" word. Yes, I said it—*skin*, underlying fat and all. Since I know I won't resist the temptation of its salty, crisp goodness, I simply

Here's A Hint

I was born and raised in the midwestern farm country. Beef was a staple. We ate chicken only occasionally and fish rarely or after one of our trips to Canada to fish for northern pike. So rather than cut out beef altogether, I have learned to use it in moderation. *Gradually* replace beef meals with chicken, fish, or vegetarian meals. When you do cook beef, broil or bake it. Aren't crazy about it that way? Try grilling it on the barbecue or get an inexpensive grill that sits on top of your stove. It doesn't have the charcoal flavor, of course, but it grills the meat nicely, giving the outside the same crusty texture of the barbecue while it lets the fat drip off. Or try this: brown beef in a pan sprayed with a non-stick spray, then cover with beef broth and vegetables such as onions, peppers, and tomatoes and simmer until done. It will be a real taste treat. Remember, to make it low fat, you must purchase cuts as low in fat as possible. Ask your butcher for a recommendation or look for cuts with as little marbling as possible. For "gravy," add a little cornstarch to the juices after you drain or lift off the fat with a spoon. Cook until slightly thickened and pour over meat or stir fry. Get adventurous—try herbs you haven't tried for a new taste treat and ENJOY!

cook skinless, boneless chicken breast most of the time. I save whole poultry for special occasions. When I roast a turkey for the holidays, you can bet I'm going to skin that bird for myself before it ever hits the dining room table! A beautiful, brown, whole turkey, set on the table for pop to carve? In this house, not a chance! Make your choices. Cut out what you want to, cut down on what you won't give up.

Now, the first part of *Lifestyle Sculpting* we've discussed. That was the use of the STOP Plan to start losing weight. Become aware of your eating and begin turning food down when you aren't hungry or in serious need of comfort food. Use a journal. Write about what you are feeling or work out your frustrations by cleaning the house or raking leaves while you cuss out the neighbor, husband, boss, or kids. But don't eat, *do* something. Burn off that feeling—don't bury it in the kitchen. We'll discuss this more under stress management, but first let's start sculpting your eating habits.

Here's A Hint

Weight Loss Myths

1. Don't eat after 6 p.m. **Wrong!** Eat when you need to. If I eat dinner early, before 6 p.m., for instance, then I will snack and/or eat all evening, guaranteed. If I postpone dinner until around 7:30, I am not hungry again before I turn in at 9:30 or 10 p.m.

2. Have a big meal at noon instead of in the evening. **Wrong!** At least if you are a food addict. A big lunch can send you around the bend. Large lunch for me? Sure, I can do that. It lasts from around noon until bedtime! Better to eat lightly until the evening meal and then compulsive, food-addicted eating behavior is not triggered.

3. Don't snack between meals. **Wrong!** Eat when you need to. If you are hungry, eat a fat free snack, whether it's a handful of pretzels, salad, fruit, or fat free cookies.You will satisfy your hunger and when lunch rolls around an hour later, you won't be tempted to eat everything, including your plate, because you are starving.

RULE #1

IGNORE EVERYONE'S ADVICE, INCLUDING MINE, IF IT DOESN'T WORK FOR YOU. Listen to your own body, your own signals. Don't listen to the typical diet myths unless they fit your personal situation. Learn to know the difference, using what works for you and discarding all the rest.

Food Changes - Step One

Phase One in the sculpting process is to make changes you can easily live with. Remember, do things in small phases. Yes, it will take longer, but it will last! **STEP ONE** is to make simple minor changes. Go from whole milk to 2% to 1% to non fat. Take time to adjust your tastes in between. Use one kind of milk for several weeks or a couple of months before you change it again.

My husband grew up on a ranch drinking the cream from the top of the milk pails. He now enjoys 2% and can even handle 1% on occasion, although I still haven't been able to give him skim milk.

Use skim milk cheeses, low fat cottage cheese, or experiment with the new fat free varieties. Some are quite tasty, depending how you use them. Many companies now have fat free or reduced fat desserts that are excellent. Keep in mind if you are in one of those needy phases and eat a whole box of fat free or low fat cookies, you are still way ahead of the game by not eating a whole box of cookies loaded with fat. So for Step One, replace several foods you use frequently with low fat or non fat varieties. Just these few simple

Here's A Hint

Many times we are not satisfied by the food we eat because it is too plain or unexceptional. By using the herbs you can dress up fish or chicken or vegetarian dishes so that you will enjoy using them more often as you decrease your intake of beef and pork.

If you really have the urge to eat fried food, try this for a substitute:

Take fish or chicken and cut into strips about 3/4" by 3". (I use red snapper but any firm fish will do.) Roll the strips in egg white or non fat milk and then in seasoned Italian bread crumbs. Place on a pan sprayed with non-stick spray and bake at 375 degrees until done. Fish usually takes about fifteen minutes and chicken about twenty-five or thirty. Just be sure fish flakes and chicken is no longer pink.

Add to that "fried" finger food, oven fried potatoes. Cut peeled or unpeeled potatoes the size of french fries. Place on sprayed baking sheet and brush with a minimum of melted low fat margarine. (Non fat margarine does not cook well!) Sprinkle with salt and pepper, seasoned salt, chili powder, garlic salt, or whatever spices you like. Bake at 375 degrees, turning once or twice, until tender. Usually twenty to thirty minutes.

Ready? Sit back, put your feet up, and (shhh - eat in front of the television if you want to) and chow down on your low fat "fried" food. Once your tastes have adjusted to these lower fat recipes, you will enjoy this version of your old favorites so much that when you do eat fast food restaurant fries or fish, you'll taste and feel the fat in your mouth. You will find this kind of "fried" food enjoyable and guilt free!!

changes had my weight moving down fairly rapidly. When I hit a plateau that lasted several months, it was time for Step Two.

Food Changes - Step Two

STEP TWO is reality time. When I designed this phase, I had hit a plateau that would not budge. I wasn't gaining weight either, but I just stayed put. It seemed like my feet were set in concrete. So I dug out the nasty bathroom scale, bought an excellent electronic food scale, and started counting. I measured and weighed everything I put into my mouth. I called this process my reality check. What was I *really* eating? I kept track of my activities. I was eating an average of 1,500 calories a day, 30% fat, and staying moderately active. Obviously, for my genetic make-up and age, it wasn't enough. So the choice was mine. Do I make more changes or am I happy at this weight and at this level of health and fitness? I wasn't, so it was time for more sculpting. First, I put the scales and the measuring spoons back in the closet, and then I started again.

Here's A Hint

Plan - Plan - Plan

Do not be caught short, tired from a day at work or chauffeuring children, with no time and few groceries in the fridge. That will send you to the corner pizza parlor for a million calories and a zillion fat grams! If you know you have a long day ahead, leave a cold supper ready to go in the refrigerator or a meal that can be zapped in the microwave. Have healthy, low fat or fat free items ready to munch and handy in case it takes you a little while to get dinner on the table.

Plan ahead and be ready! That includes going out for a meal. Have a good idea what you will eat before you walk in that door and don't be swayed by your friends. Plan your choice ahead if you know the menu that will be available and then don't look at the menu. Place your order without being tempted by all those entrees. You can do it. Just plan ahead and use the STOP Plan when you are tempted!

Food Changes - Step Three

STEP THREE is to base your next changes on your reality check. For me, that meant changing to high fiber, high bulk foods and a further decrease in high fat foods. I sat down with my journal and made a list of what I would give up. I decided to eliminate meat at breakfast (I grew up in a meat-three-times-a-day family) and to eliminate meat from most lunches. If I am dying for bacon and eggs, I have it for supper and that is the only high fat food I have that day. I am careful not to do this more than once or twice a month, if that.

I still occasionally have a meat sandwich for lunch, but if I do, I eat a vegetarian or low fat dinner that evening. Beef and pork I won't give up, but I will cut down. I eat mostly chicken and fish and occasionally have red meat.

My other concession is to cook beef or pork in as healthy a way as possible. Throw your frying pan out or learn to use it by frying with a little lemon juice, chicken broth, or water. You can stir fry or saute' just as well with those items as you can with oil. Poaching chicken and fish in lemon juice with

Here's A Hint

I don't know about you, but I'm a dessert person. I've always loved sweets and remember well the times my uncle baked cream puffs or made bread pudding. It was sheer heaven. Now I steer clear of the old favorites as much as possible, at least in that form. I sometimes make bread pudding using more bread and less custard. I switch the whole milk for skim and add extra vanilla to change the focus of taste from the egg to the vanilla. I sometimes also add egg whites and decrease the number of whole eggs by one.

Another dessert I love, and my family enjoys too, is a fat free cake. You can get these mixes at most supermarkets and they are quite good. In order not to sabotage the fat free cake, I ice it with a glaze instead of "real" icing. I use confectioner's sugar mixed with non fat milk and flavorings. This is then spread over the cake and refrigerated before serving. I add vanilla, mint, or chocolate flavorings or orange juice for a change of pace. On the orange one, I sometimes poke little holes in the top of the cake before glazing and then add glaze and allow it to soak down into the top of the cake. Don't forget that old standby, pineapple upside down cake. Make it with a fat free white or yellow mix. Use low fat margarine instead of butter in the pan with your brown sugar and pineapple (packed in juice of course) and you have a lower fat version of an old favorite.

For any of these hints that call for milk, here's a mini-hint!

If milk bothers you or you are allergic to it, try the low fat or fat free non dairy mixes. I use fat free Mocha Mix on my cereal, in coffee, over fresh fruit, and anything else I would use milk for. It's tasty and fairly low in calories plus it has no fat!

basil or dill brings out wonderful flavors as well. I also have cut my mayonnaise to low fat varieties at this point. I don't go completely fat free on this because I just don't like the taste, but I compromised and I use low fat mayonnaise in moderation. I also cut mayonnaise with red wine vinegar, dijon mustard, or fat free milk to make it more spreadable for cole slaw or pasta salads in order to use less of it.

Food Changes - Step Four

Finally, **STEP FOUR** in the food changes portion of *Lifestyle Sculpting* happens by itself, usually unconsciously. I realized one evening that I was full after dinner. I didn't want my usual low fat dessert nor had I done so for several nights without even missing it. I don't think I had missed dessert or evening snacks in twenty years.

Now I cook desserts or have fat free cakes only on special occasions. If I want something after dinner, I am perfectly satisfied with a glass of iced juice or hot cranapple tea or a piece of fruit. I have even gotten to a point where one half of an apple is enough and sometimes, even that is too sweet!

When one door of happiness closes, another opens; but often we look so long at the closed door that we do not see the one which has been opened for us.

- Helen Keller

A few years ago, I never would have believed it. But your tastes *will change* if you make the changes gradually and don't force the issue. Be sure to give yourself several weeks with one or two changes to adjust to the taste. Over time, your tastes and habits will change too. I used to eat an entire 9" x 12" pan of bread pudding in one sitting. Now I am completely satisfied with one small slice because it just tastes too rich. You will also find after several months of low fat eating that eating a high fat food will make your mouth feel as though you coated it with shortening! Just think what you must be doing to your body—yikes!

These new habits will take between five and eight weeks to establish. You can see if you make these changes gradually that it will take time to lose that weight, but it works and the changes will last. If you lose weight by *Lifestyle Sculpting*, for the first time in your life the weight you lose will stay gone—***permanently.***

A sound mind in a sound body
is a short but full
description of a happy state
in this world.

- John Locke

Health is the vital principle
of bliss, and exercise
of health.

- James Thomson

CHAPTER NINE

Lifestyle Sculpting
Activity Changes

It made me gladsome to be getting some education, it being like a big window opening.

- Mary Webb, 1800s

Now, for the second phase of *Lifestyle Sculpting*. This is the activities. Notice, I did not say "*exercise*." Yes, I exercise. But you can bet I didn't when I started. As I said earlier, if I couldn't do it on a horse (most things, anyway), I didn't think it was worth doing. So again, *Lifestyle Sculpting* comes in stages.

Activity changes - Step One

STEP ONE is simple. Get off that couch or out from behind your desk. Start by taking a short

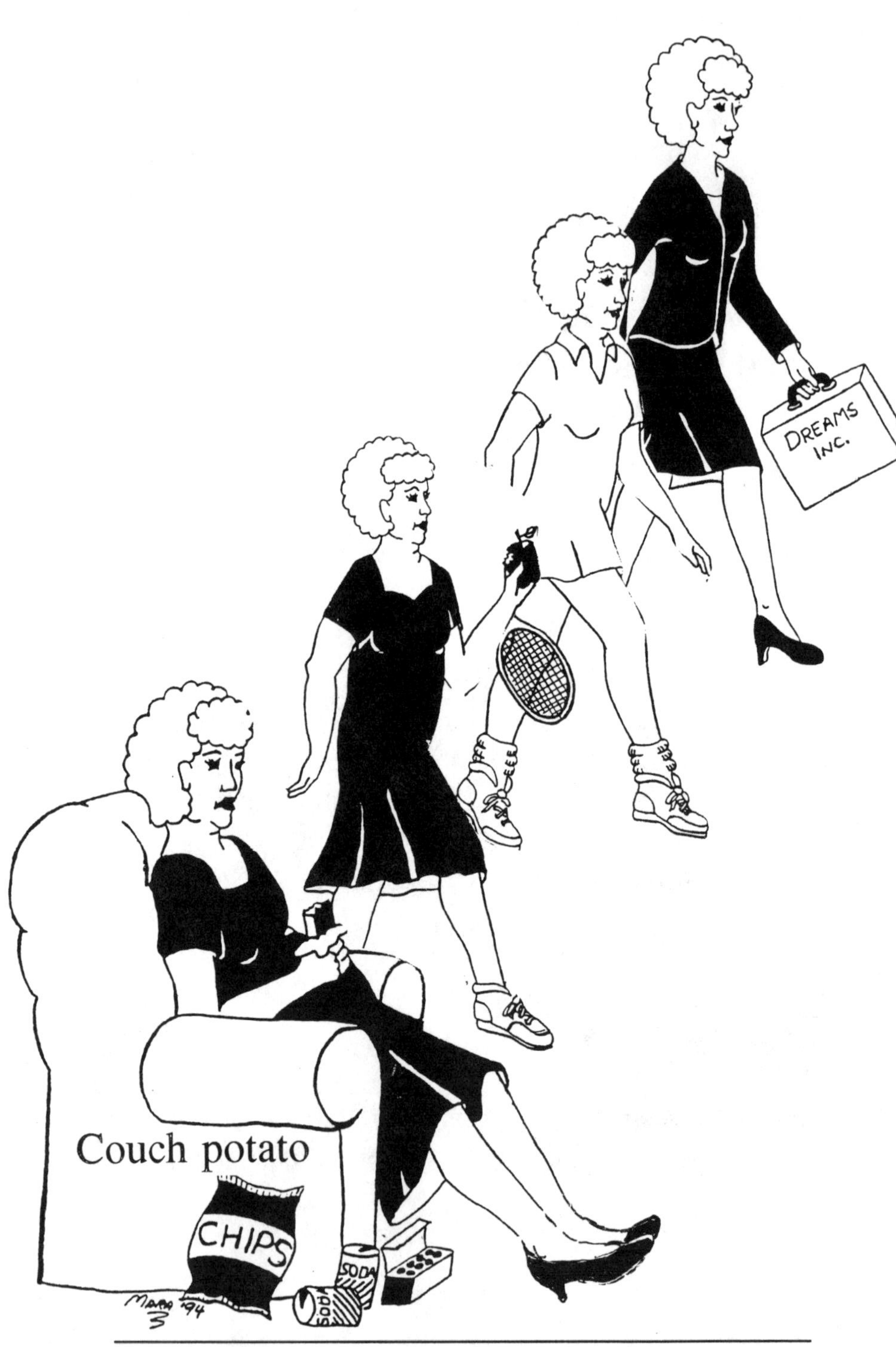

Couch potato

stroll during your coffee break and don't take it over to the donut box! Get some co-workers to go along or go alone and enjoy fifteen minutes of peace and quiet—whatever best suits you. Find something of interest to do other than regimented exercise. Have you always wanted to learn to play the piano, dance, or paint? It is never too late to learn anything. Can't afford lessons? Read John-Roger and Peter McWilliams' book *DO IT! Let's Get Off Our Buts*, which I include in my Lifestyle Sculpting Kit.

Forget your "buts" and *get going*. Can't afford an activity? Offer to trade with someone else. What do you do well that you could teach them? Sewing, cooking, computers, typing? Barter! It's a great way of getting things done for nothing except your time and effort. Can't take those classes because of child care problems? Trade baby sitting with a friend so she can take a class on a night different from yours. Work it out. It's worth it.

Activity Changes - Step Two

STEP TWO sneaks up on you. You're off the couch, losing weight, and feeling better. You have more energy. Suddenly, you *want* to take

Here's A Hint

Do you have trouble getting motivated? *Get a friend enthused about your plan.* Whether you want to take an art class or a dance class, find someone with whom you can attend classes. It is much easier to cancel a lesson if you are going alone. If you have a date with a friend, have arranged child care or transportation, it will encourage you to be there! That's all you have to do—***get*** there! You'll motivate yourself after that. But if you need help to get off that couch and to get moving, *get it.* Call a friend, coworker, or a family member, **but do it**. If you just can't get anyone else charged up over your interest, call the person you are going to take classes from and ask if they have a client who might like a partner. Maybe they can create a "buddy" system in their classroom setting that would help many of their students, not just you. You might mention the added advantage to the teacher that if they work up this kind of system, they might keep students longer who would otherwise drop out if their motivation begins to wane. Decide what sounds interesting and get busy. Pick up that phone and track down a companion for this experience and then join a class, club, or whatever. *Just get off your butt and* ***go for it!***

more classes or to play with your children in the park. Forget the house (if it's basically sanitary). Your family can either survive in a messy house or pitch in and help. Get out and enjoy the warm spring days or crisp fall ones. Look around—enjoy! Do something—*any*thing.

There is a whole world of opportunities out there: arts, crafts, classes, walking, dancing, seminars, and workshops. Get a job if you don't have one outside your home and feel you have to justify being out of the house. (There's another book on that idea alone!) Get up in front of the country music station on the radio or television, *move those feet* and have some fun.

Do you have a local YMCA or YWCA? They usually have all sorts of classes, exercise and otherwise, for very reasonable fees. Oftentimes they have child care available as well.

You men out there who need to lose weight can kill two birds with one stone. Actually, *three* birds with one stone. Take the kids for a walk and give your wife time for a long soak in the tub or time in the easy chair with her favorite book.

Here's A Hint

To get started walking, I needed serious motivation. I used Richard Simmons's walking tapes and music for awhile and still do on occasion. The rhythm and music are great. For diversity, I also made some of my own. I took my purchased cassettes and then took favorite pieces from those and combined them on one tape. Motivation for me is not only music. I not only enjoy the rhythm of some of my '50s and '60s stuff, but also songs with a message. These included things like Garth Brooks's *The River* and *We Shall Be Free*, and Reba McEntire's rendition of *Respect* and *Somebody Up There Likes Me*. I also have a soft spot for gospel music and walked to the gospel music of Sandi Patti. Peace and quiet, relaxation—that meant music without lyrics such as James Galway's flute music on *The Wind Beneath My Wings* cassette, Mozart, or the *Somewhere in Time* sound track. Of course a hint of romance always holds my attention. George Strait and his *Pure Country* sound track with *I Cross My Heart* or the sound track from *Dirty Dancing* always keep me walking.

As you can see, I have diversified tastes. Cater to your own personal preferences and see what keeps you moving the best. Buy the tapes you like best and pick and choose songs from those to place on a CD or another cassette. Then—***get moving***. You can do it!

You'll do something good for both of you and spend quality time with your children at the same time. Better yet, take her out too and make your walking time a family affair.

Activity Changes - Step Three

STEP THREE is wonderful. You will be feeling much better by now and you will *want* to do more. Trust me. If you said I would *ever* walk on a treadmill and enjoy it, I would have called the men with the butterfly nets for you. But today, I walk and love it. I started by making tapes of my favorite motivational music and walking for only ten minutes a day listening to them.

As I felt better I walked faster and longer. I was getting bored with the walking, so I added working my horses. I figured if I could get fit, so could they. Now, about this time, I hit a reality check because my weight and fitness improvements stalled. I thought my weight loss would never budge again. So I sat down and thought over my options for exercise. Obviously, I love working my horses although they didn't appreciate getting fit in the least. And, I have to admit to myself and to you that I was enjoying walking to a certain extent by then.

Few people can fail to generate a self-healing process when they become genuinely involved in healing others.

- Theodore Isaac Rubin

What I needed was diversion. I was beginning to be bored by the treadmill. So I moved it into the living room despite the "lovely" decor that created so that I could watch my favorite old movies on the VCR while I walked. I have always been a sucker for romance, be it a book or an old mushy movie. Now I watch half of an old movie classic while I walk on the treadmill, dreading the time I have to stop because I have to turn off the television. I don't let myself watch the second half of the movie until I am back on the treadmill.

Also, when I am finished with any exercise, I treat myself to a long soak in a huge bathtub (my husband *swears* that is why I bought this house). I take a crystal glass filled with iced juice or mineral water with a twist of lime, into the bath with a romance novel or a good mystery and relax and let my muscles get the benefit of the hot water. This is just about my favorite time of the day.

Still not enthused about exercise or classes? Volunteer. Help is needed in nurseries, hospitals, senior centers, shelters, day care centers, and food banks to name just a few. Give of yourself, of your own personal expertise. You and society will reap the benefits.

It is easy to live for others;
everybody does. I call
on you to
live for yourselves.

- Ralph Waldo Emerson

You'll be up and moving, learning, meeting new people, and experiencing life while you give to others.

I can hear the excuses from here. No time, no money, no baby sitter, physically unfit, and so on and so on. It's the biggest case of "buts" I've ever heard. Well, I was in all of those boats and used all of those "buts" myself. I worked, was a graduate student, had adult children and grandchildren, was on a tight budget, and have a minor heart problem. I did it anyway and so can you.

Tackle your road blocks one at a time. First, you are your most important consideration. You and your health. Selfish? Not in the least. If you must insist on taking care of everyone else, consider this. *How can you do that if you aren't healthy?* Make time for yourself and your *Lifestyle Sculpting*. You *deserve* it.

Money tight? There are all kinds of ways, like the bartering I already mentioned. You can use junior college classes, classes for seniors, women's programs. Many companies now have excellent wellness programs for their employees. Buy

Here's A Hint

Not a physical fitness junkie? Probably not if you need *Lifestyle Sculpting*! I sure wasn't (and still am not). Don't set yourself up for a fall by setting out impossible goals—better yet,don't set any goals at all! If you are sedentary, there are very few of you who will successfully jump cold turkey into a fitness club, aerobic workouts, and daily sessions with a personal trainer. Believe it or not, that is what it takes for many television and motion picture stars to keep their twenty year old figures when they are thirty, forty, or fifty. They have tremendous motivation—their careers depend on it. If you don't have a driving desire and need to do this, it won't work.

Do you remember a few years ago when Richard Dreyfuss did a movie called, **What About Bob?** Dreyfuss played a psychologist/author who wrote a book called ***Baby Steps***. That is exactly the premise you need to apply to your own personal fitness. Literally take baby steps. First, get off the sofa and walk around the house, then around the yard, then to the mail box. Ours was only one tenth of a mile from the house, but I used to wait until I went somewhere in the truck to pick up the mail! When these things are a snap (and they **will** be), *do a little more*. Get out of the house for the classes we've talked about. Join a women or men-only gym if you are not comfortable with the thought of attending a co-ed facility. Do one low-impact aerobics class a week. No, you won't get the full benefit of doing aerobics once a week that you would if you did them four or five times a week, but you just started. As that one class gets easier, attend a second and a third. We all learned to walk and then run by using baby steps. Apply the same thing here. *Get going* **now**. Take that first tiny step of your choice and I promise, more will follow soon.

equipment on credit if you have to. Join the YMCA or the YWCA. There is always a way. Physical problems? Check with your physician and start slowly. If you're too heavy to stress your legs or are physically challenged and in a wheelchair, just get active in classes. I know it isn't easy to get out and about in these cases, but you can do it.

What about starting an exercise support group with others in your condition? Perhaps you can seek the help of the community center and local exercise or physical therapists in setting something up. If you are able to, sit in your chair and move whatever you can move. *Any* movement is an improvement over just sitting.

Remember, sculpt in stages. When you are more active and feeling better, do exercises with your arms while you read or sit in the living room. Watch a favorite program and keep your arms moving, lift your legs, anything to get moving. There is equipment available to help you exercise with bad backs, bad knees, etc. Just look around and see what is available to you. When you first

Age is opportunity no less
Than youth itself, though in another dress,
And as the evening twilight fades away
The sky is filled with stars,
invisible by day.

- Henry Wadsworth Longfellow

start, take very short walks around your house or yard. You will be surprised at how the time you spend will increase as will the intensity of the activity because you feel better and begin to enjoy it.

One last comment on activities—*age*. Don't let that stop you. My husband and I have taught horseback riding to people of all ages who have never been on a horse in their lives. Older people learn to ride, bike, ski, and many other activities. In our community, we have quite a network of tennis-playing seniors.

People take up dancing, swimming, and hiking in their later years every day. If you have always wanted to learn to do something special and your doctor agrees, do it! *It's never too late.* If you don't have a group in your age bracket and experience level for a special activity in your area, run an inexpensive classified ad in your local paper. Ask for others with the same interest to contact you or the local community center to encourage them to offer a wider range of activities. You might be amazed at how many responses you get from others interested in the same things you are.

Growing old is no more than
a bad habit which a busy
man has no time to form.

- Andre' Maurois

As you increase your activities, you will observe several things. You will lose weight, not only from exercise but from these non aerobic type activities themselves. It's rather difficult to feed your face when you are playing the piano with both hands or holding a palette in one hand and a paint brush with the other. Your stress level will be lowered as your interests in other matters grow.

As they grow, you will broaden your horizons, leading to a *richer*, *fuller,* ***healthier*** life. Both your physiological and psychological well-being will improve.

Get busy. *Now.* Today! Put the book down and walk in circles around your living room for five or ten minutes. Just *move*! Then come back and read some more.

Look to your health; and if you have
it, Praise God, and
value it next to a good conscience;
for health is the second
blessing that we mortals are
capable of; a blessing
that money cannot buy.

- *Izaak Walton*

CHAPTER TEN

Lifestyle Sculpting

Stress Management

Rule #1. Don't sweat the small stuff.
Rule #2. It's ALL small stuff.
- Unknown

Finally, *Lifestyle Sculpting* requires some changes in how you manage stress. We need to look at personality traits that give you trouble as well as environmental pressures that can cause stress. If you are not sure of the source of your personal stress, seeing a psychological counselor can prove beneficial. Most of us, if we sit down and think about it, know what is bothering us—whether it's the job, the kids, an unhelpful spouse, or whatever. The question is, how do you recognize these stressors and how do you cope? You have to accept that facing problems head on and getting them out in the open cannot possibly be worse than stuffing your emotions down with a chocolate mousse.

Happiness depends upon ourselves.

- Aristotle

Stress Management - Step One

STEP ONE. First, take a look at your personality traits. These fall into the hotly debated "Nature versus Nurture" discussions. Were women *born* to be nurturers or were we *taught* to be? Are we born perfectionists or do we learn it at home? Does it matter where we got it? I say **"no."** The result is the same regardless of the cause. We suffer from the *"ought tos"* and the *"should haves"* **big** time.

You men, too. I know there are plenty of you who take care of your family, provide a roof, and three square meals a day, not only because you want to but because you *should.*

I want all of you to condition yourself to send up a red flag every time those words flit across your consciousness. I want the red flag going up like a rocket at dawn. You are going to re-train yourself to respond to **"I want"** and **"I need,"** not *"I should."* **Period.** That's it. No excuses. You do what you do for your family and your career because you want to and you enjoy it. If not, *stop doing it.* Something has to change. Don't do anything simply because you think you should.

The man who never alters his opinion
is like standing water, and
breeds reptiles of the mind.

- *William Blake*

Stress Management - Step Two

STEP TWO. The second step is looking at your self-esteem or self-love. It is a very important element in good mental and physical health and it is also a key element in successful, permanent weight loss. Self-love is not narcissistic. You can love yourself and hold yourself in high regard while still caring about the needs of others.

But you're important too. You deserve to be looked after, to eat well, to have time for outside interests. As you practice Lifestyle Sculpting, you will begin losing weight, have more energy, and feel better about yourself.

Figure Four has a short quiz that addresses your level of self-esteem. Take the quiz and see where you fit in. Are you answering "no" more often than "yes" to the questions? If so, then you may need to work on improving your self-image and self-love. The research I did on obesity showed a very strong correlation in lowered self-esteem in those of us with weight problems.

Figure 4
Self-Esteem Check

1. Do you say what you think rather than what people want to hear?

2. Are you happy with yourself, content with who you are and what you do?

3. Do you believe so strongly in certain values that you defend them regardless of what others think?

4. Do you feel equal to others, neither superior nor inferior?

5. Are you concerned with the needs of others, sensitive to needs other than your own?

6. Do you enjoy yourself whether you are at home, working, or just relaxing?

7. Do you have confidence in your ability to deal with problems and crises?

8. Do you feel comfortable acting on your own best judgment regardless of what others say?

- continued on page 170

I'm betting you need help here just as I did. *Figure Four* has some suggestions for improving this. Work on the ideas there and make a concerted effort to re-evaluate your own worth. Remember to send that red flag sailing up when you hear yourself saying "should."

You're **not** crazy. You don't need a *(shhh,* not too loud) mental health professional. *Please!* There is nothing wrong with seeking advice on any health issue, physical or mental. There are several levels of support out there.

Many support groups are available in most communities. Our little town of 2,000 even had a women's center where women could get together and talk about their concerns. Support groups are generally focused around specific concerns and interests such as problem teens, drinking problems, cancer survival, or any other common concerns.

Also excellent are the psychological counselors. These professionals generally have a master's degree in psychological counseling and a great deal

Figure Four *(cont'd)*
Improving Your Self-Esteem

A common problem with low self-esteem is setting goals that you cannot reach and then chastising yourself when you "fail." A place to start then is to set *small*, achievable goals with which you can be happy. Praise from others won't help; we usually do not trust this feedback. So if you are facing a major project, break it down, do it in stages, and give yourself credit for a job well-done at the completion of each phase. Use this program as a place to start. Make one, and only one, food change for instance. When you successfully do that you will gain courage and faith that you can accomplish more. Make another change, again only one, and when you have done that, give yourself another pat on the back and continue.

Honesty is an issue here. Look at yourself with clear, honest vision. Do you care about others? Are you honest and forthright? Do you work hard for yourself and your family or for your company? Give yourself some slack. You are okay and you need to accept that. It is not wrong to believe you are good at what you do and be proud of it. Develop a sense of pride in what you accomplish and who you are. Take a look in the *Recommended Reading Appendix* for more information on this very important topic.

of experience dealing with all sorts of family, marital, and employment issues. Generally, counselors of this type will focus on what is causing your current problem and on ways to deal with it.

There are of course psychologists and psychiatrists. Therapy with these professionals can often be very costly and time consuming. In some cases, they tend to dwell on the past, looking at causation rather than offering management techniques for today. Be sure to get the level of help and therapy appropriate for your concerns. If you try a counselor and your personalities don't mesh, switch. There are many good ones out there and you have the right to try several until you find one with whom you click.

As we move into the 21st Century, it is becoming more acceptable for men and women to seek some outside help with stress management and mental health issues. Simply having a neutral party listen to you talk about your concerns is enough to lighten the load. Whether you use counseling to deal with a crisis such as a death or divorce or whether you use it to improve self-esteem, it is

*The greatest happiness is
to know the source
of unhappiness.*

- Jyodor Mikhailovich Dostoevsky

*To have known how to change the
past into a few saddened
smiles—is this not to
master the future?*

- Maurice Maeterlinck

worth it. Once you take advantage of this assistance, you will fall back on it to deal with most of your life transitions. It smoothes the way for easier transitioning and a healthier emotional lifestyle.

Stress Management - Step Four

STEP FOUR deals with your environment. Environmental influences play a huge part in being overweight. We've already discussed these somewhat under causation. What we need here are ways to deal with these issues.

Things such as stressful jobs, a family that is less than supportive of your efforts or needs, peer pressure, and many other outside influences can cause you difficulty. Again, getting some counseling can help with these.

Attending seminars and workshops on stress management can also offer many helpful hints on dealing with these stressors.

One major way to deal with stress caused by those around you is simple. People treat you the way

Here's A Hint

Having a great day? Feel thinner? Take a photo of yourself, then note the date and circumstances. What is it that is making you feel great even if you are still heavy? Do that all during your journey. Whether you feel like you have lost weight or not, a little or a lot, take the picture and note why you are feeling special. When you are finished, you'll have a photographic record of your passage to good health. You'll also have a record of what makes you feel special so you can repeat those experiences.

you *teach* them to. That's right. If Johnny talks to you like you're dumber than dirt, you taught him to. Hold on now. Think about it. You have *allowed* it or he wouldn't do it. Same thing if the boss treats you like a peon. It's up to **you** to take control and let these other people know you will not tolerate being treated in such a way.

As you both demand and give respect to others, you will be amazed at how they will begin to see you and how you will see yourself. Car sales people can be a perfect example in many cases. You go to a used car lot and come out feeling like you have been run over by a steam roller. No more.

Walk into that place and when a sales person approaches, you lay out the ground rules as soon as soon as he arrives. "I'm looking for a car. I want information, not hard sell. I will deal with you and only you, not your superiors and everyone else in this place. Can we do business like that or shall I take my business to the dealership down the street?" Maybe that seems rude, but it isn't. You can be cordial and friendly while still having a "Trust me—we're doing this my way or not at all" attitude.

I have discovered that we may be in some degree whatever character we choose. Besides, practice forms man to anything.

- James Boswell

Be firm in your expectations and give the person a chance to deal with you correctly. If he or she doesn't, ***turn and walk away.*** Do *not* allow that person to bulldoze you. The same applies to teens or spouses who demand their own way, or your boss, or your overprotective mother. You do not allow that any longer. Teach them how you expect to be treated and be firm. No backsliding. Your self-esteem will leap up considerably, you'll be proud of yourself, and feel great. All of that will help you in your *Lifestyle Sculpting* for permanent weight loss and those other people will respect you far more than they did when you let them walk all over you. You deserve better than being a doormat. *Demand* it, kindly but firmly today.

So, for emotions and stress, if becoming aware is enough to make you better, fine. Use the STOP Plan to make yourself think about what you are doing and why. For instance, if the kids are pushing you to go to a movie you don't believe is suitable and you are caving in, work the STOP Plan. Before you open your mouth to say yea or nay, STOP. *Think* about why you are reluctant for them to see the show or why you are reluctant to see it.

To be obliged to beg our
daily happiness from others
bespeaks a more lamentable poverty
than that of him who
begs his daily bread.

- Charles Caleb Colton

Consider your OPTIONS. If you believe the movie is truly not a good one, can you compromise by taking them to a better picture that you will all enjoy? If you don't give in because you know you have made a healthy choice for your children, will you be happy? Will you feel remorse if you give in?

After looking at these options and the consequences of your decision, then PROCEED. Do what you believe is best. Be firm. Stick to it. As children, spouses, or strangers begin to learn that you think before you respond and that you do things for specific reasons, they will accept your decisions and the fact that once made, you will not go back. Use the program in the same way if you are angry about something. STOP, THINK, look at your OPTIONS (why are you responding this way and is it your best choice?), then PROCEED with your choice of action—not someone else's.

The STOP Plan, worked consistently and correctly, should go a long way in helping with stress management. If becoming aware of what motivates your stress helps but isn't enough, then

We honor ourselves and our friends when we can tell them how we feel.

- Theodore Isaac Rubin

you can see a counselor, read up on the subject (see *Recommended Reading Appendix*), or track down some workshops on stress management.

Do not ignore the stress problem. Without viable solutions and ways to deal with stress, you will be working the STOP Plan frequently to stop your grazing. Change your immediate response to anger (or any other stressor) from a food binge to a call for an open forum on the problem or scribbling in your journal and you will need the STOP Plan less and less often. *Lifestyle Sculpting* in this area will replace the reflex of reaching for food with a far more healthy reflex of reaching for a phone to call the offender or picking up your pen to write.

Now that we have looked at food, activity, and stress management changes, we have one last hump to get over. I call it the *Mega-Plateau*. The one on which you feel nothing short of an Act of God will get your weight moving down again. It's time for *Truth or Consequences*.

Lying to ourselves is more deeply ingrained than lying to others.

- Dostoevsky

Chapter Eleven

The Final Plateau—Truth or Consequences

Saddle your dreams afore you ride 'em.
- Mary Webb, 1800s

Here it is—the **Mega-Plateau**. You have slammed into it with the power of an eighteen wheeler hitting a concrete buttress at eighty miles per hour. Nothing you seem to do is making any difference. Your weight has stabilized and won't budge. You are still above what you consider your healthy weight to be.

Don't get depressed or anxious about this plateau. Everyone, and I do mean *everyone*, hits this. It is nature's way of letting your body stabilize and adjust to the fewer calories, greater activity, and dropping weight. Your body thinks something is wrong and will "shut down" the weight loss systems to protect you from starvation. It takes time to adjust, but if you persist in the program, your weight will begin dropping again. Just know

What man wants is simply
independent *choice,*
whatever that independence
may cost and wherever
it may lead.

- Dostoevsky

when you hit the Mega-Plateau, it is **not your fault**; it isn't anything you are doing wrong. What it means is that you will need to step up your efforts in the areas of food monitoring and physical activity in order to get off that plateau and get your weight sliding down again. This is also a good time, if you have stayed at one weight for quite some time and believe you are working your STOP Plan and are still *Lifestyle Sculpting*, to give some serious thought to your choices.

This is a good time to face the truth or accept the consequences. Do you really want to lose more weight? Be brutally honest with yourself. It will do you no good to kid yourself. Are you working the STOP Plan and *Lifestyle Sculpting*? I mean, really working them? Are you eating anyway and choosing to ignore the STOP Plan, cramming food down your throat without giving yourself time to STOP? Remember, *Lifestyle Sculpting* offers real choices for real people.

Are you choosing to eat too much? Have you gotten a little too attractive for your peace of mind as you shed those pounds? Are you feeling

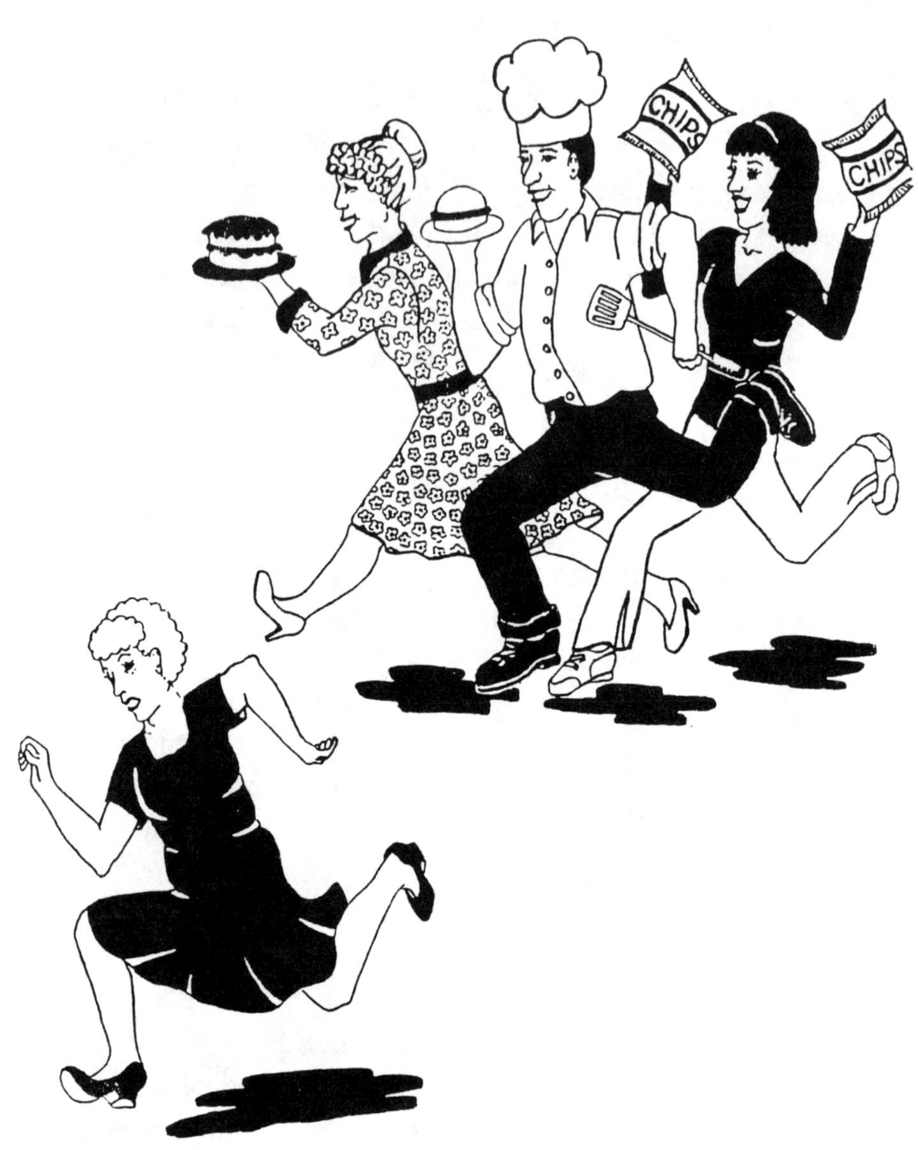

SABOTEURS

insecure and vulnerable, wanting to hide behind those old layers of social insulation (fat)? Think and think some more. Re-read this book from start to finish. If you decide that you need to or want to stay a little heavier than what might be physically healthy in spite of what you tell yourself about wanting to be thin, look at your choice with a high powered microscope. If you need help here, get it!

Don't let yourself deliberately wipe out the healthy changes you have made. Is the comfort food really more important to you than the weight loss or can you do something else to comfort yourself? If the food is more important to you, then you need to take another long, hard look at why you want to lose and if you truly do want to lose. See what is going on in your life that is sabotaging your efforts.

There is no blame here. I'm not trying to say your weight is your fault or shame on you if you decide to stay heavy. But I want you to remember that staying a little heavier than you think you "should" is your choice. If you need that protection, if you enjoy the food you are eating and just plain don't want to cut out anymore, that's

Here's A Hint

Visualization

Now don't get excited. I'm not going to ask you to get "new agey" on me. But positive thought is a very strong force. If you believe you will not lose weight, *guess what??* You *won't!* If that is what you think, you are carrying around an image of yourself as fat in your brain and that is what your subconscious will pick up on. Even though your mouth is saying you want to lose weight, your inner self sees a picture of your "fat" image and gladly complies with your requests. Get a picture of yourself, slim and healthy, not unrealistically gaunt, in your mind instead and keep it there! Visualize yourself as you *want* to be. See yourself slim and healthy. *Believe* you will be thinner, and you *will!*

okay. You are an adult. The choice is yours to make. But don't hide behind excuses. It is okay for you to say, "I'm happy the way I am and I'm staying at this weight. If and when I want to lose more, I will make the choices necessary to do that."

Your weight is no one's business but *yours*. Make your choice. If you choose to remain moderately active and make no more lifestyle changes, then accept that you have made that choice and do not feel guilty about it.

Maintenance. I hate that word. It implies that you will slide back into old ways and pack that weight back on. That is a very real possibility. In fact, I guarantee it if you dieted off the pounds.

However, if you have done your *Lifestyle Sculpting* correctly, which means slowly—one step at a time, you won't have a problem with maintenance unless you choose to let those old eating habits and inactivities-from-hell back into your life.

At this point then, all you need to remember is to remain aware. It is easy to get careless. If you

We lie the loudest
when we lie to ourselves.

- Eric Hoffer

start nibbling or grazing, STOP. Use the STOP Plan every time you reach for food and carefully assess what you are doing and why.

If you haven't already gotten a refrigerator magnet with the STOP Plan on it, copy the cartoon in this book and tape it to the fridge, the dashboard of your car, the closet, bathroom mirror—anywhere that you hide and sneak food.

Is it just time to tighten up? Have you gotten sloppy or is something going on in your life which needs talking about to the family or to a counselor?

Don't sabotage yourself. Be aware of what you are doing. We all know that we can feel when we have gained a pound or two or when we are losing it. Think!

Saboteurs are everywhere. Use the STOP Plan to guard against the invasion. *Lifestyle Sculpting* gives you the tools to saddle your dreams and to ride them to success. The *Do It! Let's Get Off Our Buts* book recommended in the Appendix and

Here's A Hint

As you can see from this chapter, remaining aware of your eating is very important. You can do several things I have discussed if you think you are getting sloppy. Hang copies of the Stop Plan drawing everwhere! Use any other illustrations which move you in the same way. **THINK** before you eat! Write in your journal, notebook, or on the table napkins. Think about why you are grazing and allowing yourself to ignore the Stop Plan.

If you purchased a *Lifestyle Sculpting Kit*, you have a "touchstone" in the form of a Stop key chain. Carry it in your pocket or snapped to your waistband—anywhere you can get your hands on it and play with it during difficult times. My touchstone was a medal I won in college. I wore that thing around my neck on a long chain and when I wanted to eat, I played with it instead. I probably drove people crazy, but I sat with that medal in one hand and the chain in my other and ran it up and down the chain! I couldn't eat because I didn't have a free hand and the medal reminded me that if I could achieve that, I could achieve permanent weight loss. Use the touchstone from the kit or better yet, get something of importance to you. Pick out anything that makes you feel good about yourself. Use it like a "worry" stone and carry it everywhere. Feeling the urge to eat? *Grab that thing and play with it!* Hold onto it for dear life. It *works*. You'll gain strength and confidence in yourself if you take time to do that and slow down long enough before you eat to work the Stop Plan.

included in the *Lifestyle Sculpting Kit* is a wonderful addition to this program to teach you how to reach those dreams. Combine the two and go for it! You can do it by getting off your butts and your **"buts."**

If you are having a serious experience with the Mega-Plateau and just cannot seem to get things moving again, reassess your dream. I highly recommend (if you haven't gotten that impression by now) the book I just mentioned. If you read this work, you will be able to more carefully define your own personal dreams. If weight loss is truly one of these, then go back to the STOP Plan and *Lifestyle Sculpting* and make your choices in order to reach that dream.

After achieving your own personal healthy state, use the STOP Plan only as needed when you feel yourself getting sloppy. You can keep the weight off and hang onto that dream for a lifetime.

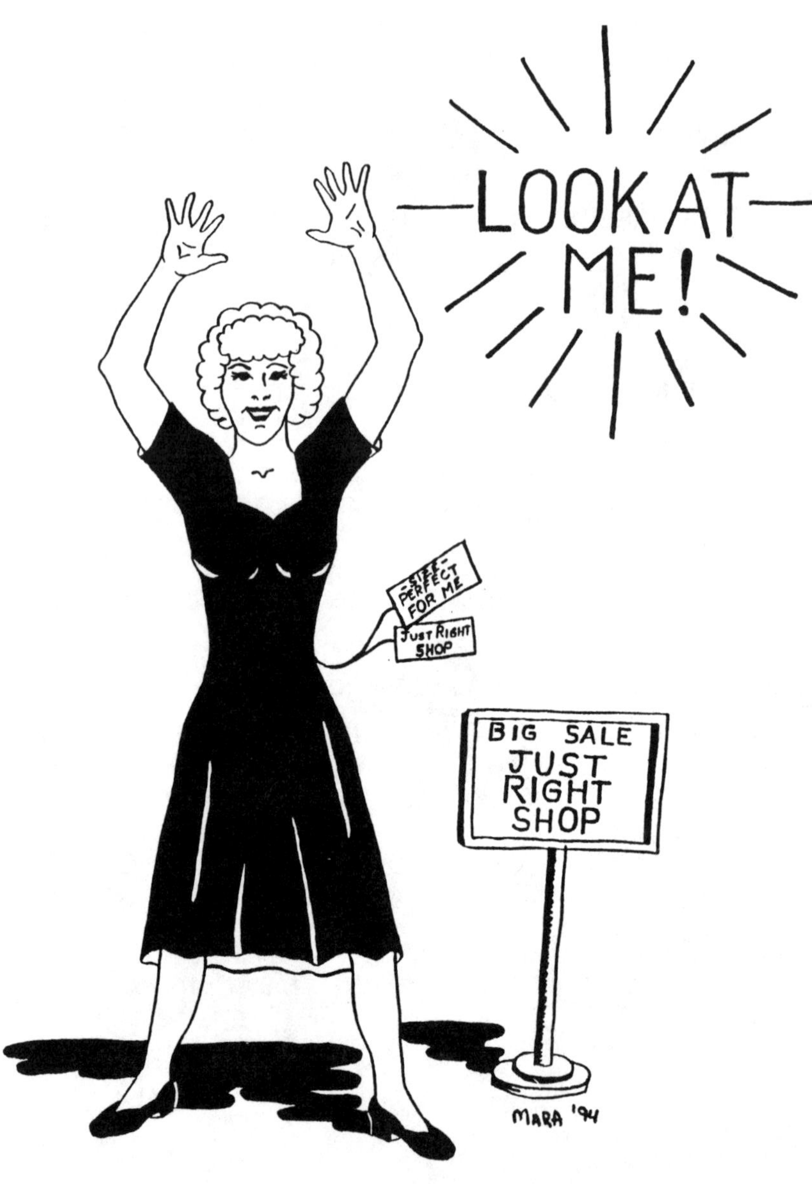
LOOK AT ME!
-SIZE-
PERFECT FOR ME
JUST RIGHT SHOP
BIG SALE
JUST RIGHT SHOP
MARA '94

CHAPTER TWELVE

Are You Ready For Success?

Our greatest glory comes not in never falling, but in rising every time we fall.

- Confucius

Another silly question, this woman asks! Is that what you're thinking when you read the title of this chapter? If I weren't ready to lose weight, would I be reading this book while I'm munching on a bag of potato chips?

As you can see from the previous chapter, not everyone who undertakes weight loss is ready. Why you want to lose it is a crucial factor in your level of success. Nothing, I repeat—nothing, not even Lifestyle Sculpting, will work for you if you are trying to lose weight for the wrong reasons.

Doing it to "earn" a new car or wardrobe or doing it to please your spouse, parents, or kids won't cut it. You have to do it for **you**. For *your* good

When we are unable to find tranquility within ourselves, it is useless to seek it elsewhere.

- Francois de La Rochefoucauld

health and fitness. Not to be attractive, not to fit some societal image of the perfect woman or man. You must do it to feel better and to be happy with yourself based on your own standards and your own personal best.

Weight loss goals are out! Don't set any goal for the number of pounds you want to lose in a week, a month, or a year. Don't even *think* about it. You will simply succeed in driving yourself crazy.

There should be only one goal for *Lifestyle Sculpting*—to feel better tomorrow than you do today. That means eating healthy, sparking an outside interest (or two or three or four), and having more energy with each passing day. That should be your goal. You will have to fight those temptations as fiercely as an evangelist fights demons.

You will be tempted to climb onto the diet carousel with every quick and easy scheme you see on the front page of a supermarket tabloid. You'll

FIGURE FIVE

Are You Ready For Success?

1. I accept that losing weight with a reduction diet will never work permanently. Y N

2. I am losing weight for me, to feel healthy and to have more energy. Y N

3. I accept that the weight must come off slowly if I want to maintain the loss. Y N

4. I accept that I am worth it. Worth any extra planning or trouble needed to succeed. Y N

5. I am losing weight for me, not because anyone else told me I should. Y N

6. I am now able to tell people what I believe, not necessarily what they want to hear. Y N

7. I am willing to get off the couch and get active. Y N

- continued on page 200

be tempted to fast or diet just long enough to make your weight start down again. *Don't do it!* It isn't worth it and it will not work. Stick to your *Lifestyle Sculpting*.

Do a reality check if need be and be sure you aren't grazing (*sly grazing*, my husband calls it) or fooling yourself about what you are actually eating and doing. Then decide if you want to cut something else out or cut down. Eliminating one thing or decreasing the size of one meal can make the difference.

My final plateau had lasted for months and I began getting discouraged and sloppy. Simply doing a reality check, tightening up again, adding one activity, and cutting back on my breakfast portions had the weight falling off again. The choice was mine. I had plenty of breakfast and it worked. I was happy, full, and energetic.

Figure Five has some questions for you about your level of readiness. Take the quiz. Be honest. If you aren't ready, you will only damage your

FIGURE FIVE (CONT'D)

8. I have accepted the fact that I may be a genetic draft horse and will be the healthiest person I can be, not what society views as thin and beautiful.
   Y N

9. I believe that the resulting weight loss will be worth "giving up" certain high fat, high calorie foods for less fattening varieties. Y N

10. I believe that if I have more good days than bad, I will lose weight, however slowly it may occur.
    Y N

All right—here we go again with the more good than bad. Do you have more "Yes" answers than "Nos"? You do? Great! You are ready. Get to work on your *Lifestyle Sculpting*; success is just around the corner. More "Nos" than "Yeses"? Take a good look at yourself and re-read the book. Are there some areas where a counselor or friend can help? Work at those "nos" until you get more "yeses" on your side and then **GO FOR IT!** *Lifestyle Sculpting* is for you.

health by losing weight and gaining it back one more time. Whether you have just started to sculpt or whether you are on your own personal Mega-Plateau, being honest on this quiz can keep you from making a disastrous choice. If you are not ready, take a long hard look at your motives.

When you are ready, and *only* when you are ready, use every resource at your disposal. Use everything you can. Put every weapon into your arsenal, but remember, the primary responsibility is **yours**.

No one can make you lose weight. No one can do it for you. ***You*** choose your course, choose which resources to use, and choose which foods to eat.

So, use this book, and I do mean **use** it. Mark it up, highlight it, dog-ear the pages if something moves you. Copy the drawings and hang them all over your house or car.

The great enemy of the truth is very often not the lie—deliberate, contrived, and dishonest—but the myth—persistent, persuasive, and unrealistic.

- John F. Kennedy

Do whatever it takes to make the *Lifestyle Sculpting* system work for you if you believe you are ready to lose that weight once and for all.

Take advantage of the counseling or support networks available to you if stress is a major element for you.

Write to me in care of: *Sierra Vista Publications, P.O. Box 1899, Sierra Vista, AZ, 85636-1899* if I can help or just to let me know about your progress.

Use your own spiritual beliefs—whether they encompass God, Mother Nature, or Whatever/Whomever you hold dear. **But**, as you face this battle, remember the Russian proverb which says, "Pray to God, but keep rowing to shore."

Good luck and good health!

Losers visualize the penalties of failure. Winners visualize the rewards of success.

-Robert Gilbert

APPENDIX A

Recommended Reading

Food & Nutrition

Regret for the things we did can be tempered by time; it is regret for the things we did not do that is inconsolable.

- Sidney J. Harris

APPENDIX A

Recommended Reading

Food & Nutrition

This section of recommended reading includes books on nutrition, cooking, and the physiological influences behind food responses. These are all books I have used over the years. Although those that mention specific diet plans did not work for me, they all have some interesting information. If you are particularly interested in how the body works and interacts with food, these should help. The cook books have some wonderful recipes. Thin eating does not have to be boring or tasteless as you will quickly see if you try some of these recipes.

HERE'S A HINT

I repeat throughout this book that fat is more important than calorie counting. You do not want to spend your life worrying about calories. As you learn which foods are naturally low in fat, you will simply choose more of those than ones you know to be high in fat. A good average is to eat foods with lower than 20% fat calories most of the time. To figure that out, use the following formula.

Say a food has 90 calories per serving and 1 gram of fat. Each gram of fat has 9 calories. You multiply 1 x 9 and get 9. Then divide the 9 calories of fat by the 90 calories per serving. That will give you 10%. You know then that the food you are about to eat is only 10% fat calories, well within your limit.

Try another one. You have a food at 225 calories per serving and 8 grams of fat. Multiply 8 x 9 = 72. Divide 72 by 225 (32%). This one is well above your 20% ideal so work your Stop Plan and think before you eat it! But if you want it (especially if it is half an avocado), then eat it! Just don't do it often.

BELLERSON, Karen J.

1993 *The Complete and Up-To-Date Fat Book.* This is a guide to fat and calorie content in more than 25,000 foods. As you know by now, I am not interested in the calorie count other than its relation to the fat. Concentrate on low fat or fat free foods. Use this book to check high fat foods, then work the STOP Plan and make your choice to eat or not! Ms. Bellerson even has a little pocket version out now that you can throw in your purse or brief case.

BENNION, Lynn J., et al.

1991 *Straight Talk About Weight Control.* This book is quite academic. It is rather heavy and detailed but it has excellent information on the physiology of obesity. It also addresses American culture and eating disorders. Some very interesting reading if you want in-depth data on the problem.

Look to this day poem

Look to this day,
For it is life,
The very life of life
In its brief course lies all
The realities and verities of existence,
The bliss of growth,
The splendor of action, The glory of power -

For yesterday is but a dream
And tomorrow is only a vision.
But today, well lived, makes every yesterday a dream of happiness
And every tomorrow a vision of hope.
Look well, therefore, to this day.

- Sanskrit proverb

HELLER, Rachel and Richard.

1991 *The Carbohydrate Addict's Diet*. Excellent reading on the physiological processes of food addiction. Drs. Heller and Heller give valuable information regarding hyperinsulinemia and how to know if you are carbohydrate addicted. This book could help you pinpoint food triggers if you have not confirmed what sets your eating binges off. The doctors have also put some nice recipes in the back of this one.

HILL, Lynne S.

1987 *The People's Nutrition Encyclopedia*. An excellent reference for fat and calorie counts. Again, pay particular attention to the fat, not the calories unless you are comparing the two to see what percentage of fat you are getting. See the sidebar on the opposite page for more on this.

Strength is the capacity to break a chocolate bar into four peices with your bare hands—and then eat just one of the pieces.

- Judith Viorst

KIDUSHIM-ALLEN, Deborah.

1981 *Light Desserts, The Low-Calorie, Low Salt, Low Fat Way.* This is an older book but it may be in your local library. The recipes are delicious and if you are anything like me, desserts can be your downfall at first. As I have said, my tastes have changed but I do still enjoy a really rich dessert. There is a great recipe for caramel flan in this one!

LEVIN, Allen Scott, M.D.

1983 *The Type 1/Type 2 Allergy Relief Program.* This is an older book, but it is an excellent one. It is well worth a used book store or library search. The information in this one tells you how to accomplish a rotational allergy diet. This allows you to test one kind or family of foods at a time in order to find just which ones you are allergic to and how your body reacts. There is excellent information in the book about how your body reacts to various allergens by causing headaches, breathing problems, water retention, or many other physiological manifestations. I believe this one is no longer in print, but, as I said, well worth looking for.

A good meal ought to begin with hunger.

- French Proverb

ORNISH, Dean, M.D.

1993 *Eat More, Weigh Less.* I have included this book for the wonderful, gourmet recipes it includes. There is a collection of 250 of them - so experiment, have fun, and enjoy good eating! The book also includes some good information on the importance of eating in a culture and of eating during stressful times. Dr. Ornish talks about "soul" food and nourishing your mind to nourish your body. Good reading!

PISCATELLA, Joseph C.

1991 *Controlling Your Fat Tooth.* Excellent information on how your body reacts to fat and how to decrease your cravings for fat. The book includes an important section on the dangers of having a high fat diet. The book also includes more than 200 recipes by Bernie Piscatella that are quite good.

*Habit is habit, and not to be flung
out the window...but
coaxed downstairs
one step at a time.*

- Mark Twain

PRUDHOMME, Paul.

1993 *Fork In The Road.* Wonderful book with great recipes! Everything from the ordinary (done in extraordinary ways!) like macaroni salad to the gourmet-like shrimp and artichoke salad. This marvelous chef includes great desserts and old favorites cooked in a low fat manner, like oven fried catfish. Buy this book, try the recipes, and good eating!

SIMMONS, Richard.

1990 *Deal-A-Meal Golden Edition Cookbook.* This book is filled with inspiration and delicious recipes. Richard adds a few poems and childhood memories that are touching to those of us who have been fat. The book doesn't give nutritional analysis since the book is intended for use with Simmons's Deal-A-Meal program, but since he espouses low fat cooking, one assumes the recipes are in good shape. He does give an analysis of how they relate to his program which will give you an idea of the equivalents of the foods like bread or meat.

One thing life taught me—if you are interested, you never have to look for new interests. They come to you.

- Eleanor Roosevelt

Motivational Books

No one tests the depth of the river with both feet.

- Ashanti Proverb

Motivational Reading

On the following pages are just a few of the books I found to be inspirational.

Reading them will both uplift and entertain you as you pursue your new path to radiant health.

An afternoon in a library or bookstore will turn up many, many more books that you can turn to again and again for motivation. Trust your instincts—the books that are right for *you* will make their way into your hands.

When you are tempted to eat, feast on these instead!

If you have formed the habit of checking on every new diet that comes along, you will find that, mercifully, they all blend together, leaving you with only one definite piece of information: french-fried potatoes are out.

- Jean Kerr

MCWILLIAMS, John-Roger and Peter

1991 *Do It! Let's Get Off Our Buts.* As if you haven't heard enough about this one! But I cannot recommend this book strongly enough. It is a fabulous, motivational work that will set you on the straight path to your dreams. These two authors will teach you how to define your dreams and how to pursue them in spite of your "buts." I am including this book in my *Lifestyle Sculpting Kit*, but if you don't want or need the kit, go to your local bookstore or library and get this book! You won't regret it. The authors have other books out too. One is *Life 101* and another is *Wealth 101*. These are also motiviational and have the same easy reading, informative format.

POWTER, Susan.

1993 *Stop the Insanity*. Well, if any of you don't know who Susan is, where have you been? You can't turn on the television in the morning without hitting one of her infomercials or go to the market without seeing her face somewhere. This book is as great as she is. While Susan goes

Discouragement promotes inaction, and inaction guarantees failure—a life of not living our dreams.

-John-Roger and Peter McWilliams

a bit overboard in my humble opinion on avoiding fat, she is enthusiastic and the kind of lady many women need to look to for guidance. You tell people what you think they want to hear? Listen to Susan. She is a dynamo. She says what she thinks and she takes no prisoners. She's funny and entertaining and on the right track for weight loss, taken in moderation. She has a wonderfully motivating story to tell and she has developed some great low fat recipes. This woman is a pistol and a great motivator. Read and enjoy this book.

SIMMONS, Richard.

1993 *Never Give Up*. This is a wonderful book filled with motivational stories from Richard's years of helping others. The book also contains some of his poems about eating and weight loss. The book may bring a few tears to your eyes as you recognize your own struggle with weight in these case histories. But look at the outcomes—these people made it and so can you!

The wind-footed steed is broken down in his speed, whilst the camel-driver jogs on with his beast to the end of his journey.

- Sa'di

Appendix B

Recommended Tapes

The person who makes a success of living is the one who sees his goal steadily and aims for it unswervingly. That is dedication.

- Cecil B. De Mille

APPENDIX B

Recommended Tapes

You will notice that in this section, I have listed only a handful of tapes. That is because, as I already told you, I hate to exercise. I have included only the tapes that worked for me, the worst exerciser in the world! I know there are others out there. If you are into exercise or as you get more so and your energy increases, try the different ones at your local library before purchasing a zillion tapes you may not like. Many tapes are too fast or advanced for the more uncoordinated types like me. So borrow the tapes whenever possible and try them out before buying.

There is only one set of aerobic tapes that I use with any regularity. These are the Richard Simmons's, *"Sweatin' To The Oldies"* tapes. I love old music, especially that of the fifties and sixties. These tapes are geared to those of us who are obese, not to slim little models who want to stay slim! The moves are easy to learn and the music, especially if you grew up on it, will really keep your toes tapping and your body moving. *"Sweatin' To The Oldies 2"* is my favorite. This one includes floor work for muscle toning. Even

Perseverence is more prevailing than violence; and many things which cannot be overcome when they are together, yield themselves up when taken little by little.

- Plutarch

if I don't do the whole tape, I use this portion to strengthen my arms and legs and to warm up before I get on the treadmill or go out for a walk.

Richard also has a wonderful tape out for stress management. This one is all stretches, set to classical music. He does no talking on this one, simply leads you through a relaxing routine set to beautiful music. This is very rejuvenating and is a great way to start and/or end your day. Called *"Stretchin' to the Classics,"* this is a lovely tape.

For technique, no one can beat Susan Powter's, *"Abs and Oils."* She does an excellent tape showing the proper form needed to do a workout. So many tapes just have you moving, hustling to music. Susan shows you the correct way to work, which makes a tremendous difference in how effective the workout is. She also provides information on fats and cooking without them which is helpful. My favorite part is her emphasis on correct movements, though.

Also on my short "favorite list" is a tape by Cheryl Tiegs called, *"Super Shape-up Program."* This is a good tape for beginners because it is interval training. Cheryl mixes low impact aerobics with toning exercises at one or two minute intervals. For those of you not in good shape, this will keep your heart from working too hard and will also help you tone muscle.

Regret for the things we did can be tempered by time; it is regret for the things we did not do that is inconsolable.

- Sidney J. Harris

Remember the hidden benefit of more muscle—it burns more calories than fat does.

And speaking of fat, for information on fit versus fat, try Covert Bailey's, *"Fit or Fat For The 90s."* Good information on losing fat and getting fit. For those of you who don't know Covert Bailey, he is entertaining while being informative. An excellent speaker, he is fun to listen to although he does get into the physiology of fat a little deeply for some.

Finally, for toning, the *"Abs of Steel"* and *"Buns of Steel"* tapes are good toners. They are not for beginners. When you get into your program and are feeling better, give these a try. You can learn good exercises and positioning but keep in mind these people are **fit**. Do just a few repetitions and do not overdo it! But the tapes have good information and for someone like me—who doesn't know diddly about exercise, I learned a lot from them.

Remember, if you have been sedentary and are overweight, check with your doctor before leaping into any heavy exercise programs! Your heart is a muscle and if it hasn't been worked, it needs to be conditioned just like your arms or legs. ***Do not overdo it right off the bat.*** Take your time and start *slow*. You can and will build up and do more than you ever thought you would.

Success is not the result of spontaneous combustion. You must set yourself on fire.

- Reggie Leach